STORIES ALLWAYS

"tales for children's well-being"

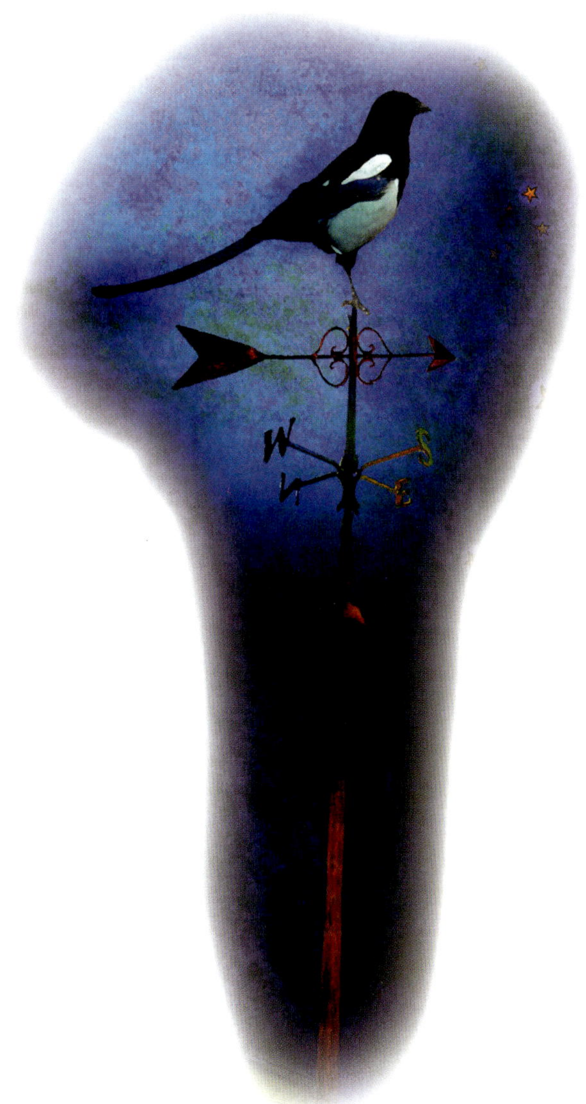

By Ruth Kirkpatrick • Illustrated by Catty Flores

A Storytelling Resource Pack

ISBN: 978-0957-463-905
Printed and Published in Great Britain by Stories Allways,
North Lodge, Glencorse House, Penicuik, Midlothian EH26 0NZ, UK
Tel: (+44)1314451507
E-mail: ruth@storiesallways.co.uk
Website: www.storiesallways.co.uk

Published: November 2012

All illustrations including cover by Catty Flores.

Typesetting by Tenacious Ltd, North Finchley, London N12 0DA
Printing by Abbey Print, Dalkeith, Midlothian EH22 4AD

British Library Cataloguing in Publication Data applied for.

Ruth Kirkpatrick has been a social worker since 1986, specialising in child protection and then social inclusion in education. From 2003 to 2006 Ruth was a development worker for Scotland's child welfare organisation, Children 1st, with special expertise in storytelling. She is a trained Gestalt counsellor.

In 2006 Ruth founded 'Stories Allways', which offers training courses in storytelling and runs story-based programs in educational, mental health and community settings. Ruth has worked in schools, prisons, and children's residential centres.

Although based in Scotland, Ruth works throughout the UK and abroad, designing and running storytelling projects. She has been a guest storyteller and trainer at international festivals.

Ruth lives near Edinburgh with her husband, two daughters, and a dog and pony.

ACKNOWLEDGEMENTS

In some cultures, they say that it takes a village to raise a child. It feels to me as if it has taken a town to produce this pack! No list can do justice to everyone who has contributed to this package. But to all whom I have met on this story road, and who have helped by thought, word or deed, I am truly grateful. I have been blessed with so many generous, talented people who have influenced and helped me, including:

Claire McNicol, the spark, for making all seem possible. "Boldness has magic, power and genius in it. "

David Campbell for his wisdom. "I've taught you all I know and still you know nothing."

Stanley Robertson, Duncan Williamson and Sheila Stewart. "When you drink from the stream, remember the spring."

Donald Smith and all at the Scottish Storytelling Centre for inspiration, support and encouragement over many years.

Pam Anderson and Bob Skeldon for believing in me. "They are rich that have true friends."

Catty Flores for perfect illustrations.

Richard Holloway for his kind words.

Robbie Robertson, Linda Williamson and Cathlin MacCaulay for much-appreciated permissions and encouragement.

Jenny Coles for caring and careful editing. "An oak is not felled at one stroke."

David Pringle for invaluable production guidance and for proofing.

Haydon Farrar and Andrew Philp at Tenacious for creative and super-efficient type-setting.

All at Abbey Print for prompt printing.

Jenny Gardener and Gica Loening for their wonderful talents. "It's about more than the music."

Angus Lyon and David Gray for patient recording sessions and smooth CD production.

Scott McDonald (cdflyers.co.uk) for speedy CD Pressing.

Bambie Maxwell for laughter and love. "Old friends and old wine are best."

Roni for extra voice, eyes and ears, and for everything – I couldn't have done it without you.

My daughters for their priceless feedback and advice.

My parents, sisters and extended family for their constancy and love. "The apple never falls far from the tree."

Last, but never least, my thanks to all the children who inspired this pack with their praise and their honesty, their hunger and enthusiasm, and by being themselves. "May the road rise up to meet you."

For

My dear Jack Sprat, Roni, and our girls Sula and Sylva.
"She that has love in her breast, has spurs in her sides."

and

My parents, my first and best storytellers.

TABLE OF CONTENTS

Preface ix

Introduction 1-5

Using this Pack 6-12

Key to Activity Symbols 13

1. The Legend of Beira and Bride 14
- Introduction 14
- Story: 'The Legend of Beira and Bride' 16
- Activity 1: Story Soundscape - *Music* 20
- Activity 2: Make a Creation Myth - *Storytelling* 22
- Activity 3: Woven Snowflake - *Art* 23

2. The Taen Awa 24
- Introduction 24
- Story: 'The Taen Awa' 26
- Activity 1: Baby Care - *Social Skills* 30
- Activity 2: Make a Waterfall - *Music/Movement* 32
- Activity 3: Story Map - *Art/Storytelling* 34

3. Finn McCool and the Young Hero's Children 36
- Introduction 36
- Story: 'Finn McCool and the Young Hero's Children' 40
- Activity 1: Arruchica - *Movement* 46
- Activity 2: Story Soundscape - *Music* 48
- Activity 3: What are You Best at in the World? - *Social Skills* 50

4. The Seven Ravens 52
- Introduction 52
- Story: 'The Seven Ravens' 54
- Activity 1: Story Sticks - *Art/Storytelling* 58
- Activity 2: Story-making with Objects - *Storytelling* 60
- Activity 3: Give a Blessing - *Social Skills* 61

5. The Cockerel and the Sultan 64
- Introduction 64
- Story: 'The Cockerel and the Sultan' 66
- Activity 1: Envelope Puppets - *Art/Storytelling* 68
- Activity 2: Story Sticks - *Art/Storytelling* 69
- Activity 3: Story Soundscape - *Music* 71

6. Jack and Marigold 73
Introduction 73
Story: 'Jack and Marigold' 75
Activity 1: My Hero - *Social Skills* 81
Activity 2: Anyone Who - *Movement/Social Skills* 84
Activity 3: Harvesting a Story - *Storytelling* 86

7. One-Eye, Two-Eyes, Three-Eyes 88
Introduction 88
Story: 'One-Eye, Two-Eyes, Three-Eyes' 90
Activity 1: Letter Writing for Emotional Literacy - *Social Skills* 95
Activity 2: Re-telling the Story - *Storytelling* 97
Activity 3: A Special Place - *Art/Social Skills* 98

8. Tatterhood 100
Introduction 100
Story: 'Tatterhood' 103
Activity 1: My Hero - *Social Skills* 108
Activity 2: Personal Stories - *Storytelling/Social Skills* 110
Activity 3: What's Behind the Door - *Storytelling/Art* 113

9. The Dog and the Peacock 115
Introduction 115
Story: 'The Dog and the Peacock' 117
Activity 1: Customise a Candle - *Art* 119
Activity 2: Let's have a Ceilidh - *Storytelling/Social Skills* 121
Activity 3: Group Poem - *Social Skills* 123

10. The Good Goodbye 125
Introduction 125
Story: 'The Good Goodbye' 127
Activity 1: Design a Cloak - *Social Skills/Art* 129
Activity 2: Group Poem - *Social Skills* 130
Activity 3: Give a Blessing - *Social Skills* 132

Sources 135-137

List of CD Tracks 138

PREFACE

I first met Ruth Kirkpatrick in a women's prison. I was there to present a BBC Radio Scotland programme on an initiative called 'Story Book Mums and Dads' that was being tried out in the prison. Behind the project was a tragic fact: all over Scotland children were going to bed at night knowing their mothers were not at their bedsides telling them stories as they sank into sleep, but locked away in distant cities. So why not get the mothers to record stories onto CDs which the children could listen to as they cooried down to sleep at night? Thus the programme was born. It was heartbreakingly successful, and we heard of children so happy to hear their mothers' voices that they played the stories to themselves over and over again.

To help launch the programme, Ruth was invited to come to the prison in question and tell the inmates a story. I have to admit I was a little bit wary of this part of the procedure. We'd be up against some pretty hard-bitten characters, I mused, and it's anyone's guess how they would respond to this young woman spinning them a tale. I needn't have worried. One prisoner in particular caught my eye. She was standing at the back looking bored out of her mind, shifting restlessly, clearly wanting to be somewhere else. As Ruth spooled out her story of the Seven Ravens I kept my eyes on that tough young woman lounging against the wall. I saw her attention slowly being caught, then I watched as she became transfixed by Ruth's story, her mouth opening wider and wider as the tale took her over; and I realised with a pang that she had probably never been told a story in her life, never been taken out of herself with the magic of the narrator's art.

Ruth Kirkpatrick is one of Scotland's most dedicated and compelling storytellers and in this volume and accompanying CDs she has brought together the best of her art to help other storytellers keep this ancient skill alive. The main thing a great story does is to open us to the wonder of existence and its challenges and complexities. Like the best folk music, the greatest stories come out of the deep memory of the race. They are the way we have made sense of the joys and sorrows of life, and they take us back down the years to the oral tradition that is at the root of our best art. These old stories have been kept alive by people like Ruth who have inherited them and handed them on enriched with new layers of meaning. It is absolutely characteristic of the storyteller's vocation that Ruth has chosen to make this fund of stories available to others. There's a moment in Alan Bennett's great play *The History Boys* when Hector says to his pupils of great poetry, '...pass it on boys, pass it on...'. That's what Ruth is doing here: she is passing on to the future some of the great stories of the past so that our children will be enriched and challenged by their timeless wisdom.

Richard Holloway

Richard Holloway was Bishop of Edinburgh until 2000. He was Chair of the Scottish Arts Council from 2005-2010. He is founder of Sistema Scotland, the charity that seeks to change the lives of children through music.

INTRODUCTION

"Eye to eye, mind to mind and heart to heart" - Stanley Robertson

I believe that we are all storytellers. However, some of us lack confidence or practice, or simply do not know which stories to tell. This pack may help! As human beings we are irresistibly attracted to story. Story is in all that we do, whether it is holding a conversation at a bus stop or re-telling Homer's *The Odyssey*.

One of the greatest challenges for those involved with children is helping them to lead fulfilled and happy lives. It can seem a daunting task. We need tools to assist us in nurturing children's emotional, social and physical well-being, as well as encouraging their skills in planning for life's choices, changes, and relationships. There is a growing awareness that stories can make a positive contribution to children's social education and well-being as well as to literacy. Traditional stories in particular touch on many of life's challenges and dilemmas: it is one of their great strengths and attractions.

But where can we find the best stories? This pack provides a collection of stories and activities that I have found effective through my own practice. They have successfully engaged children and young people's attention, as well as providing a springboard for discussion or related activities. The aim throughout is to promote emotional well-being and mental health in the 7-14 age group.

Why is Storytelling for me?

I am often asked how and why I became a storyteller. As a social worker, I always tried to find effective and creative ways of communicating with children. From 1999, I was part of an interdisciplinary team of social workers and teachers which was engaged in a pilot project in a deprived area. I was working alongside Claire McNicol, who had recently embraced oral storytelling. Claire was keen to try using traditional stories in a social work setting, and the project team began to experiment with stories and associated activities.

I was presented with the challenge of working with a class of nine-year-olds whose local area was undergoing demolition. They seemed distressed, and were unable to sit still, let alone listen. Moreover, the children had endured three changes of teacher that year. Eighteen of the twenty-four children were known to the Project for reasons of neglect, abuse, ill health, loss or other family trauma. I had tried all my usual strategies for engagement: talking, acknowledging, art work and drama. Nothing seemed to really reach these children behind their defences. I decided to try telling a story originally from a book by the great storyteller Duncan Williamson. Heart pounding, I told my first traditional story. This was a new experience for all of us. I was amazed at the children's response. They hung on every word, their faces at peace, their bodies stilled. Their response to being told a story was completely different to their response to talking. I knew that there was something powerful and complex, and yet ancient and simple going on.

Storytelling was taken into the Project team's 'toolbox' of ways to work with children. There was excitement as we shared stories and follow-up activities that we had found to be successful. The children with whom we worked were outspoken (and sometimes brutally honest) in their responses, which was a great way to learn.

Donald Smith, Director of the Scottish Storytelling Centre, was full of praise for the work we were doing, and suggested some mentoring from a traditional storyteller. I sought out Stanley Robertson, because he hails from the rich traveller tradition, and because, like me, he comes from Scotland's north-east. So, tape recorder in hand, I went to see Stanley.

We are incredibly lucky in Scotland to have had many custodians of the traveller tradition. While the rest of us fixed our eyes on the television and let the old songs and stories shrivel through lack of breath, the travellers have continued to gather around the fireside. Stories from the traveller tradition are vivid, rich in drama, and infused with universal themes. There are stories of love and loss, change and transformation, death and rebirth, sometimes full of tragic pathos but often leavened with humour. Stanley flowed like a river with stories, songs, riddles and games in the traveller tradition of word play. He explained that his grandmother had taught him his stories, "Eye to eye, mind to mind and heart to heart". And that is how he taught me.

Meanwhile, at the school, the children came to expect a story each time I saw them, and my repertoire grew. I used storytelling with classes, groups and individuals. I even sometimes told a story as part of 'whole family' work. I visited one family many times and felt ineffectual in the face of the circular narratives presented by the parents about their child. Eventually, I tried telling them a traditional story. This changed the dynamic of subsequent sessions.

I learned so much by telling stories, chosen to either reflect a child's situation or a contrasting experience. My work led me to one boy, Robert, who was looked after by his grandparents. The eldest of four, Robert's father had committed suicide and his mother, a drug user, lived nearby but was absent from his life. Robert was constantly in trouble at school for shouting and fighting. His concentration was poor. He struggled to make friends. I was asked to spend time with him to process his trauma and loss, and to help improve his social skills. Robert was very loyal to his mother and refused to talk openly about his feelings on any subject. He seemed to have taken the burden of responsibility for his siblings on his young shoulders. His build was small but he had a big presence. I told Robert the tale of Tom Thumb, who was also small but nevertheless very resilient. I thought that he might connect with such a character. The tale begins with a poor woodcutter and his wife longing for a child. One day the wife walks by a river and wishes on a leaping fish that she might have a child, even if he were only the size of her thumb. Robert interrupted at this point, saying angrily, "And when she got him I bet she changed her mind!" This was the first acknowledgment of maternal rejection expressed by Robert. Obliquely, under the cloak of the story, he felt safe to begin to express his feelings. This breakthrough marked the beginning of a new phase in our communication.

Why Stories?

From the beginning of time, stories have been used in raising children: to entertain and to educate, to comfort and to control. Long before writing existed, oral stories were used to pass on and reinforce beliefs and behaviour, community values and knowledge, thus influencing both societies and individuals. And so it continues today, when stories are told in many different ways – through books, radio, film, and of course television. The tradition of storytelling remains dominant.

Stories engage the attention, being full of action and emotion, and often showing how others deal with problems. Traditional stories in particular often depict characters facing obstacles and challenges or coping with adversity and hardship. The 'truth' about the issues such stories deal with is carefully dressed up in the clothing of 'story' which makes them accessible to the reader or listener. It is perhaps one reason why traditional stories have survived for so long. They 'talk' to children about universal issues - about challenge, change and loss, and about aspiration, fortitude and promise – in terms that children can understand. They offer 'maps' for ways out of situations which seem hopeless. They show children that they are not alone with their anxieties and fears, their longings and hopes.

Significantly, most traditional stories end in a place of hope, giving us inspiration. It is this element of hope which many consider to be crucial in the value of stories for children. Bruno Bettelheim says that a story told actively and with genuine feeling can

> give the child the conviction that after all his labours a wonderful future is awaiting him - and only this belief can give him the strength to grow up well, securely, with self-confidence and self-respect. (*The Uses of Enchantment: The Meaning and Importance of Fairy Tales*, Vintage Books, New York, 2010 [1976], p.156)

Many traditional stories are about growing up and finding one's place in the world. They tell of the challenges involved, but also provide clues as to how we may all reach the state of 'happily ever after' by finding in ourselves qualities such as resourcefulness, perseverance and either moral or physical courage.

Stories (and especially traditional stories) are often consigned to the nursery, to be experienced and then put away with childish things. However, I would argue that there is no better vehicle for presenting complex dilemmas of life to children, and for helping them to make sense of the world, than story.

As children and as adults, stories form the framework and structure through which we sort, understand, relate and file experience into memory. We are our stories. Because stories are structured, they give us a firm scaffold on which to build our view of the world, creating meaning and memories.

All the stories in this collection are old, and throughout their long lives have been polished by the people who told them, in order to heighten both their impact and their usefulness to listeners. Which brings us to the storyteller and the art of storytelling . . .

Why Storytelling?

Reading a story aloud to children is valuable, but telling a story creates a special rapport, a connection that derives from direct eye contact being maintained with the listener, from the inflections of the conversational voice, and from the subtle facial expressions and body language that come with the act of telling. Above all, a story is told 'heart to heart', rather than being received second-hand from an author (however wonderful) whom the child has never met.

Storytelling encourages listening skills. Listeners are motivated to hear what will happen next. One boy, diagnosed with ADHD, with whom I shared my stories, said in evaluation that he thought his listening skills had improved. Asked why he seemed able to listen to the stories so closely, he replied, "Because they were worth listening to!" This child's attentiveness was won partly by the alchemy of telling, and partly by the story itself. Storytelling also encourages talking. Many children are bursting to tell you what they think about a character or incident from a story, yet in everyday interaction may be very reserved. Even the most introverted usually have something to say. Again, this is partly because the synergy of telling and listening have already set up a 'conversation', however one-sided it may seem on the surface while the tale is being told. Moreover, stories, told orally, are like a gift to the listener, and the listener often reciprocates this gift quite naturally and spontaneously. For some children this can mark a turning point, since talking is the foundation of all literacy. Talking develops an internal voice, which then allows us to engage in learning to read and write. Another linguistic benefit of storytelling is that it builds vocabulary. By hearing the context of an unknown word children may work out its meaning, motivated to do so by their desire to understand the story, and additionally helped by subtle clues conveyed by the storyteller's voice, gestures and facial expressions. This intuitive decoding of words enhances skills in expression and communication.

Storytelling develops the faculty of imagination in the listener, and through engagement with an imagined world, also develops crucial skills in problem-solving, and in considering options and consequences.

Storytelling encourages positive social bonds and healthy relationships, for the story takes the listeners on a journey that is both a shared and a personal experience. Close engagement with a story helps with the development of empathy and emotional literacy. Research has shown that empathy doesn't just happen, but needs to be fostered in children and young people. If it is not, then socialisation is affected. Bullying and violent behaviour can result. By hearing another's difficulty as described in a story, the listener can empathise, and see the results of the protagonist's actions. The process enhances self-reflection and also self-expression, besides providing potential role models for how someone else has dealt with a challenge or a dilemma.

Storytelling helps the organisation and ordering of thoughts in the brain. Not only is this essential for education, but it is also crucial for good mental health. The ability to cope with stress and trauma is enhanced if a person is able to order what is happening – or has happened - in their life. The habit of telling one's own story helps a person to make more sense of experiences and events. Being the author of one's own narrative, with control over the way that the story is told, can impart a greater sense of agency. The importance to mental health of having an 'internally coherent and consistent narrative' was identified by Mary Main in the 1980s and reiterated more recently by Sue Gerhardt. Mary Main's research into attachment found that emotional security in adults was influenced more by their ability to tell their own story, than by the severity of experience they had lived through. Gerhardt's description of Main's research is worth quoting at some length:

> When adults talked about their emotional lives and their important relationships in growing up, it didn't matter whether they had a 'happy childhood' or not. Their current emotional security depended more on having an internally coherent and consistent narrative than on the actual story they had to tell. The people who were in trouble emotionally were those who either found it difficult to talk freely about their feelings,

> or those who talked too much in a rambling and incoherent way. (Sue Gerhardt, *Why Love Matters: How Affection Shapes a Baby's Brain,* Brunner-Routledge, Hove, 2004, p.53, citing M. Main and R. Goldwyn 'Adult attachment scoring and classification systems', unpubl. ms. Univ. of California, Berkeley, 1985)

Storytelling can help mental health in other ways. The process of putting feelings into words enables the left and right side of the brain to become integrated. The right brain's 'felt sense' can link with the left brain's 'verbal sense' and the result is a feeling of balance. Storytelling can be soothing and reassuring: troubled youngsters sometimes comment that they love the feeling of peace in the room when they listen to a story. The process of identifying with a story or its protagonists can also have a cathartic effect: just listening to a story can give relief, as the subliminal message that 'you are not alone', that 'you have been heard', and that situations can change and improve is conveyed. The very universality of traditional stories lends them a personal dimension which can interleave with a listener's mental or emotional state. For when a group listens to a story, different individuals will hear what they want or need in that story. It is as if each listener's life experience creates hooks in the mind, which pick up certain parts of the story in a particular way.

Why These Stories?

Teachers and social workers have often asked me to recommend stories which might be especially helpful in addressing children's emotional issues. While able to provide booklists, there seemed to be a need for a specialised collection of such stories, drawn from a range of sources. So here they are, chosen for their demonstrated potential to resonate with children emotionally, especially when they find themselves in unhappy or challenging circumstances. These tales are among my most-loved stories, and they feel like dear friends, whom I'd now like to introduce to you. I am grateful to the storytellers who have woven them with voice and pen, and passed them on.

Some of these tales have been told for hundreds of years, being respected and cherished, but also undergoing subtle adaptations as they have been handed down the generations, across countries, and between storytellers. I myself have been telling these stories for the past thirteen years, and doubtless have shaped them to suit my audiences and surroundings, rather like a cloth that is pulled this way and that. They will also have been influenced by the culture and the times in which I am living, often unintentionally, but sometimes purposefully; for example, women are included among Finn McCool's helpers!

All of these tales have hope-filled endings. I believe it is crucial to nourish children with such positive conclusions in order to build resilience and optimism. I urge you to try telling the stories, and see for yourself the sustaining and inspiring effect they can have, especially when told 'Eye to eye, mind to mind and heart to heart'.

Ruth Kirkpatrick
Glencorse
November 2012

USING THIS PACK

Who is this Pack For?

The *Stories Allways* pack is relevant for use by anyone working with children, including practitioners in the fields of Education, Social Work, Youth Work, and Child and Adolescent Mental Health. The stories and activities from the pack can be used in a classroom, in groups or in one-to-one situations. They can be worked through in a sequential way or used as an occasional resource.

The pack covers many of the areas in Scotland's Curriculum for Excellence including; Listening and Talking, Literacy, Expressive Arts, Citizenship, and most particularly, Health and Wellbeing. It also broadly covers the National Curriculum in the rest of the UK.

Stories Allways offers a way to explore and discuss issues relating to personal and social development which directly or indirectly affect children's emotional wellbeing, behaviour, learning and safety. The pack has been designed both to have broad appeal, and also to address the needs of children with social, emotional or behavioural difficulties.

In addition to stories, this pack offers complementary activities which provide auditory, visual and kinaesthetic experiences for a truly multi-sensory approach. Such an approach encourages learning that is both meaningful and sustainable.

Selecting a Story

The 'start of the story' is the moment when you choose the story. It is important to spend time deciding which story is the most appropriate. This may depend variously on the occasion, on the audience, and on your own goals for any particular storytelling session.

Each story in this pack has an introductory section which, while no substitute for reading the story itself, can be a handy guide when selecting a story, as well as a subsequent reference point and aide-memoire. The introduction to each story comprises a synopsis and brief background to the story, a list of possible themes arising from the story, and a skeleton outline of the story itself.

In choosing a story for an audience, it should be stressed that it is difficult to predict just what any individual listener will take from it. Each listener will hear whatever it is that they need or want to hear, while the person alongside may hear a quite different version. This does not matter; in fact it is because traditional stories are so rich in interpretative possibilities, and operate at so many levels of metaphor and allusion, that they tend to have such a wide appeal. They resonate differently, for different people.

A particular occasion might influence the choice of story: for example, a commemorative or farewelling event (such as transitioning to secondary school) might be marked by telling 'The Good Good-bye'. A festival might be approaching, such as Christmas, for which a story like 'The Dog and the Peacock' might seem especially appropriate. Several stories are set at particular times of year, such as May Day ('The Taen Awa'), or refer to a particular season or natural cycle ('The Legend of Beira and Bride', 'Jack and Marigold').

The size, age and sensibilities of the audience are all key considerations for the practitioner in choosing a story. Big groups might be spellbound by a large and varied cast of characters engaged on an epic adventure ('Finn McCool and the Young Hero's Children'). Small groups might appreciate the reassuring fellowship of a more homely story ('The Dog and the Peacock'). Younger children might enjoy a shorter story with antics and humour ('The Cockerel and the Sultan'), while older children might respond to a more complex and layered story ('Tatterhood'). Some stories, which lend themselves to audience participation, have an energising effect (such as 'Taen Awa', 'The Cockerel and the Sultan' and 'Jack and Marigold'), while others have a calming effect which can induce a thoughtful mood ('The Legend of Beira and Bride', 'The Seven Ravens' and 'The Dog and the Peacock').

The practitioner might also consider the personal circumstances of individuals. For example, a particular story may be chosen with a child in mind who has suffered a loss or separation. 'One-Eye, Two-Eyes, Three-Eyes', which addresses the subject of grief, might be such a story. Listening to a tale which has some resonance with a child's own situation might provide some relief and comfort to that child. It might make them feel that they are not alone in the world with their own, perhaps unspoken 'story'; it might provide an occasion to share their thoughts, feelings and fears; it might offer exemplars and hope for the future. On the other hand, it may seem like too direct an experience for a recently-bereaved child to hear such a story, and so the practitioner may decide to choose another. This decision would obviously be affected by the practitioner's knowledge of the child, and by the setting. For example, it might be inappropriate for a child to hear such a story in a big class, while a small group situation, where some sense of safety and close community has been established, might offer a haven of understanding and support. Such discussions are likely to be guided by the practitioner's judgement and intuition.

In selecting a story, it should be remembered that traditional stories tend to be many-layered and open to a wide range of interpretation and reception. This makes the stories – even the same story, used several times over – very versatile. This is fortunate, because the practitioner's goals are likely to vary from session to session, from audience to audience, and from story to story.

An important point in selecting a story is that you should, at some level, believe in it. Not literally, of course – for while these stories may not be true, they are full of truths. But a conviction about the worth of a story and its themes will be communicated.

Learning the Story

The stories in this pack may be read or told to an audience, or the accompanying CDs may be played. But ideally, these stories will be told orally, as they were always meant to be, echoing true storytelling traditions. However, practitioners may be more comfortable reading a story aloud to an audience first, and, once they are familiar with it, telling it orally.

If planning to read aloud to a group, it is still important to spend some time in preparation. Many of the suggestions for telling a story can also be applied to reading aloud. Familiarity with the story, and its moods and emotions, is the key.

In order to learn a story to tell orally, it is best to begin with one that you really like. There is no right way to tell it - just your way. In fact, re-telling the story in your own words will add conviction and expression, and lead to greater audience engagement.

Here are some tips for learning (and practising) a story.

- Read the story aloud. This has a different effect from reading quietly to yourself.
- To help remember the story, write down the main points in a list, or make a mind map diagram, or make a storyboard by drawing a series of scenes. The 'Skeleton' provided in the introduction to each story will help. Doing the 'Story Map' or 'Story Stick' Activities yourself will also help (see Table of Contents).
- Go for a walk and tell yourself the story in a light-hearted manner. Focus on the sequence of action, rather than precise language.
- Experiment with your breathing: ten deep breaths before beginning (an actor's technique) eliminates any tension or nerves. While telling the story to yourself, practice pausing, and taking time to breathe.
- Experiment with your voice, finding a timbre and pitch that you are comfortable with.
- Experiment with the natural 'light and shade' in your voice. The story, of course, carries its own light and shade, which you'll find reflected in your own telling.
- Hand gestures and markedly different voices for different characters can be effective, but are not necessary. You may find that these come spontaneously as you learn the story. But it will be your own natural voice, responding authentically to the emotions and moods in the story that lie at the heart of your rendering.
- Listen to the story told on the CD in this pack. (Nb. this suggestion is lower down the list, so that you may explore the story with your own voice first if you wish.)
- Have a go at reading or telling the story to someone who will listen. (Perhaps you can try your story on a child or partner at home.)
- When you are comfortable with the story, think about whether you want to use any props. (See below, 'Telling the Story'.)

There are many books and websites giving guidance on how to learn stories, as well as organisations that offer workshops (see Sources).

Setting the Scene

Establishing an environment and an atmosphere conducive to the telling and reception of a story is important. Setting the scene and encouraging children to enter the 'story space' is part of communicating the message to children that you have a special 'gift' – a story – to share with them. This helps children to get the most from your storytelling.

If using a classroom where the children spend most of their day, it is good to give a sense of change in the environment, both physically and symbolically. Aim to create an atmosphere of safety and containment, and of relaxed calm mingled with anticipation.

Here are some tips:

- Select an appropriate room or area, considering such factors as noise and ambience.
- A 'Do not disturb' sign on the door where the session is taking place can avoid external interruptions bursting the 'story bubble'.
- Allot space for storyteller and listeners, rearranging furniture if necessary. Be sure to sit where eye contact can easily be maintained with the audience.
- Consider seating for the listeners: children sitting in seats may fidget less, but ideally these should be comfortable. Sitting on a rug or cushions is an option for smaller groups. Rugs or blankets can define a 'story space' well.
- A cloth may be hung on the wall; or draped over the storyteller's chair; or laid on the floor or on a table (especially useful if displaying objects; see next)
- Symbolic objects representing elemental or natural phenomena (so often featured in the stories) may be displayed. These might include crystals representing the earth; or a branch, pine cone or flower to symbolise growth and renewal.
- Symbolic objects representing the stories themselves might be laid out, such as shells for a sea-faring story, a bowl of fruit for a story featuring trees, a goblet for royalty, etc. These may also be useful as props, if desired. (See below, 'Telling the Story'.)
- Dim the lights, or turn them off (although too dark a room can feel gloomy, or may lead to some children falling asleep!)

When children have been welcomed into the 'story space', a candle can be ceremoniously lit, to give a sense of warmth and light. Such preparations give clear non-verbal cues that it is time to settle down for a treat - a story! If the same preparation and ritual precedes each story session, then the children will develop a regular sense of expectation and a readiness to listen attentively.

Telling the Story

Successful storytelling is not so much about giving a polished performance with dramatic hand gestures and clever voices. If you want to use these, then you may, of course, but that is a matter of individual style. Rather, storytelling is about building relationships and making connections with your listeners. Belief in the tale you are telling will enhance the rapport with your audience. Remember, these stories are all strong: they have stood the test of time, and so you can trust that they will 'do the job'. If you are nervous, it might help to remember that, by some magical transmutation, it is ultimately the *story* that the children are listening to and hearing, rather than the storyteller.

Here are some tips to help tell the story:

- Take your time settling, and breathe deeply to achieve a calm, relaxed state.
- Make eye contact with your listeners.
- Clear your mind of distractions. If you cannot focus and connect with the story, then the children cannot either.
- Recall the emotions and moods in the story, and seek to communicate them in an authentic rather than a dramatic fashion.
- Use a pace and a rhythm that suits you. Don't rush.
- Don't be afraid of pausing! This gives you a chance to breathe, and to think what to say next. It also allows the listeners time to digest what you have already said.
- Don't worry about making a mistake.
- Most importantly, be yourself, and enjoy the experience.

The use of props is a personal decision to be weighed up during preparation. Without props, children rely on their imagination and their capacity to visualise. But props can be useful in certain circumstances. Children with Special Needs, or for whom English is a Second Language, may well benefit from the inclusion of material, visual or musical props. More generally, where children might not know what something in a story looks like – say a scythe in 'The Taen Awa', or a goblet in 'The Seven Ravens' – a prop or a picture can help. A prop might add extra interest, such as a model of a traditional ship in 'Tatterhood' or 'Finn McCool and the Young Hero's Children'. Props can be used in a representational way, such as blue fabric for the sea, or shells signifying a beach, or fruit and branches for trees. Sometimes a very defined prop – such as a puppet (e.g. for 'The Cockerel and the Sultan'), or a baby doll (for 'The Taen Awa') – can become part of the story itself. Music as a potential aid might be worth considering: a triangle or a few notes on a recorder can be used to introduce different phases of a story, or to signify the passage of time.

It is worth bearing in mind when deciding to use props that they may alter the rhythm and flow of the story, and have the potential to distract as well as to engage. The real dramatic medium for the story is the human voice.

Discussing the Story

Once the story has been told (or read), the listeners can be given a chance to talk about what they have heard. Someone may have a question or comment which they immediately want to offer. If not, an open question can be asked, such as "Does anyone want to say anything about this story?" Discussion can be encouraged by asking, "What did you like or dislike in the story?" More complex or targeted questions can be posed, but be careful not to 'overwork' the story or the magic of it can be dissipated. Asking whether listeners have 'understood' the story should be avoided, as this can undermine each individual's unique response. There is no single 'correct' message to be taken from any story, and sometimes stories just resonate with the listener in a subliminal way that defies explanation or analysis. But with practice, children will soon become accustomed to discussing a story, and will listen to each other's contributions with interest.

Following Up the Story

Each story offers three follow-up activities. These allow the listener to consider the story, or issues arising from it, in a deeper and more extended way. The activities cover a range of different aims and skills which are highlighted in the introduction to each activity. Ideally a follow-up activity will be done immediately after telling the story. However, if this is not possible and the story needs to be reprised subsequently, then the 'Skeleton' in the Introduction to each story will be a handy guide.

It has been assumed that a storytelling session will usually last for about an hour. A story might take fifteen minutes, and so most of the activities have been designed to last for about forty-five minutes. However, this can vary from story to story, and from activity to activity.

All the follow-up activities can be used for a larger class-sized group, or for a smaller group. Many of the activities could also be used in individual work with a child.

Moving into a follow-up activity should be done smoothly in order to maintain the 'bubble' that has been created by the storytelling. Being prepared, with all necessary materials laid out ready, is important. The listeners should be encouraged to stay 'within the story' during the transition to an activity. This can take some forethought. Once, after telling the story 'Annie, the Best Baker in Scotland', I invited the children to make shortbread as good as Annie's. With wide eyes they approached the table where the baking equipment beckoned. Then a teacher intervened and directed them to wash their hands. The bubble burst! If, for some unavoidable reason, a seamless transition is not possible, then reprising the story (briefly, but seeking to recapture some of the magic of the original telling) is worth trying.

The follow-up activities are sometimes interdisciplinary exercises, but broadly they come under these headings:

- Storytelling
- Social Skills
- Art
- Music
- Movement

Storytelling
Story leads to story. The best way to encourage children's own storytelling (whether written or oral) is to tell them stories. The focus in the storytelling activities is on oral rather than written skills. Children generally find this emphasis liberating. However, there is usually scope for the written medium to be introduced.

Social Skills
Stories provide an excellent springboard for social interaction. They are full of social or familial situations and personal dilemmas which children can relate to and which therefore command their attention. These exercises help to tease out some of the emotions that the stories provoke and provide ways to deal with them positively. The exercises, foregrounding both listening and talking, also promote social interaction and emotional literacy.

Art
Art activities tend to stimulate reflection and discussion: active hands can calm the mind; busy hands can make it easier to talk in a group; and creative hands can release expression. It is best to use art and craft techniques that are very simple, but can look effective. In this way self-esteem can be boosted, and children can relax during the activity, rather than worrying about the end product.

Music
Oral stories have their own music and rhythm which draw the listener in. This makes introducing music to storytelling, either as an accompaniment to a re-telling of the story itself, or as an additional activity, very easy. Some children are more comfortable expressing emotion through music (whether formal or improvised) than verbally. Perhaps this is because music can feel easier or safer than trying to find words, or because music is a language in itself, or because of the sheer atavistic pleasure of music-making. Moreover, in a group, a great feeling of cohesion can be achieved by all making music together.

Movement
The follow-on kinetic activities are designed to encourage children to move and to mix, to listen and to talk, and to cooperate. These activities are especially useful as an ice-breaker when a class or group has first come together. They are also a good re-energiser after a storytelling, especially around mid-afternoon! Mostly though, they are fun!

KEY TO ACTIVITY SYMBOLS

STORY TELLING

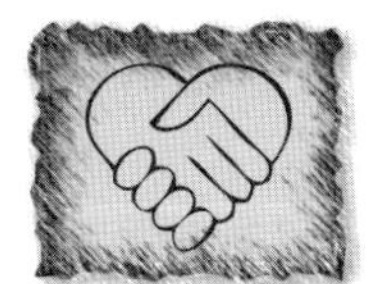

SOCIAL SKILLS

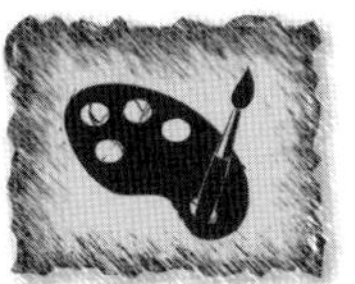

ART

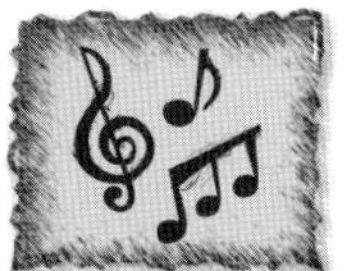

MUSIC

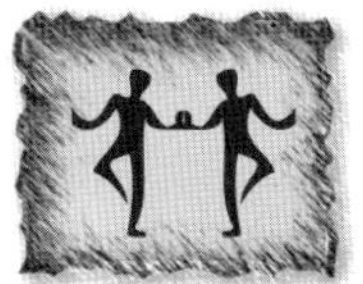

MOVEMENT

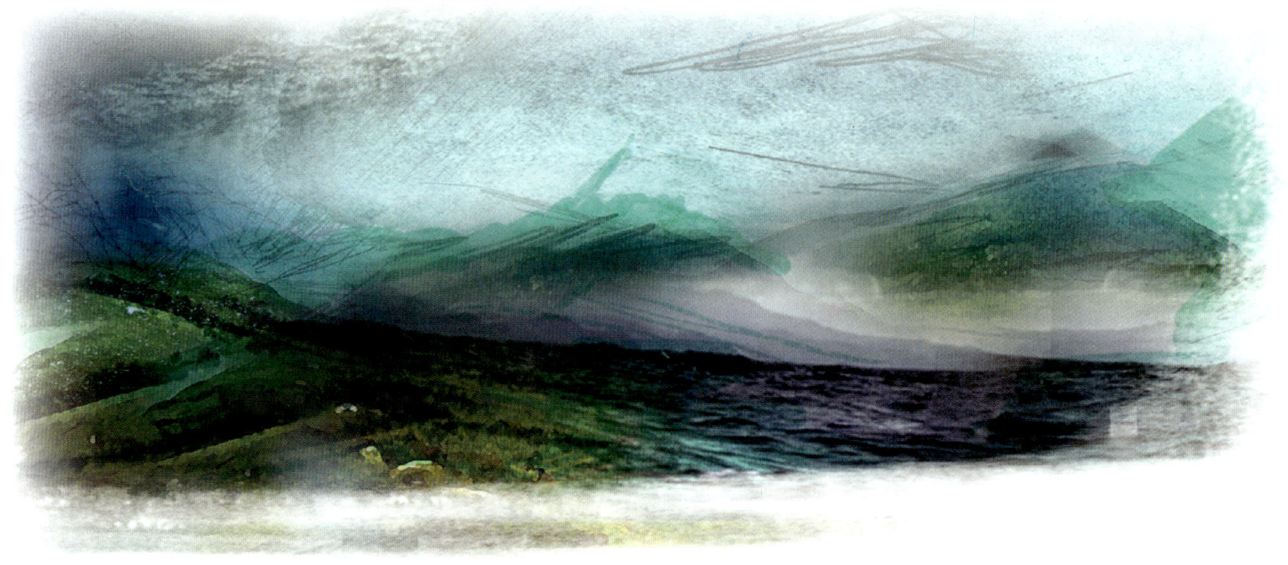

THE LEGEND OF BEIRA AND BRIDE

Introduction

Stage Primary 1 (age 5) upwards

Synopsis
This is a Celtic creation myth of how the world and the Scottish landscape were formed. Beira, the Goddess of Winter, battles with Angus Og, the God of Summer. From this encounter Spring is born. Bride is the Goddess of Spring.

Background
This story provides a suitable introduction to creation myths and Celtic mythology. It is little known but very popular when told. It is best told in the spring, when listeners can experience the battle of Beira and Angus Og as it is played out by the weather.

Suggested Themes
- The connection between people and nature
- The 'story' of the world around us and how it came to be
- The rewards of perseverance and courage, requiring hard work and a degree of risk-taking
- The power of hope, even in the darkest hour
- The power of love, even in a hostile world

Skeleton

1. At the beginning of time, Nine Maidens push a millstone and make earth.
2. Each has a creel of clay and creates the Earth as we know it.
3. Beira, Goddess of Winter, creates Scotland, the mountains and lochs.
4. She is old, lonely and tired.
5. She tries to stop the advance of spring by smashing buds and shoots.
6. Her slave, Nessa, forgets to cover Beira's well, so Beira turns her into a river, making Loch Ness.
7. While washing her shawl, Beira creates the Corryvrecken whirlpool.
8. Beira gives another slave, Bride, the impossible task of cleaning a perpetually dirty fleece.
9. Father Winter makes the fleece clean, and gives Bride snowdrops to take to Beira as a sign of the coming of spring.
10. Beira sets out to halt the advance of spring.
11. Angus Og, the God of Summer, falls in love with Bride and determines to rescue her.
12. His father, Dagda, warns him of the wild February weather.
13. Angus asks the God of August to move three of his days to February, creating 'The Days of Bride'. Angus sets out to search for her.
14. Angus and Bride marry, thus making Bride the 'Goddess of Spring'.
15. Beira and Angus clash and do battle across the skies.
16. Angus wins and spring arrives in late March.
17. Beira goes to the Summer Isle and sleeps until Halloween when she will awake, return to the mainland and reign as Goddess of Winter.

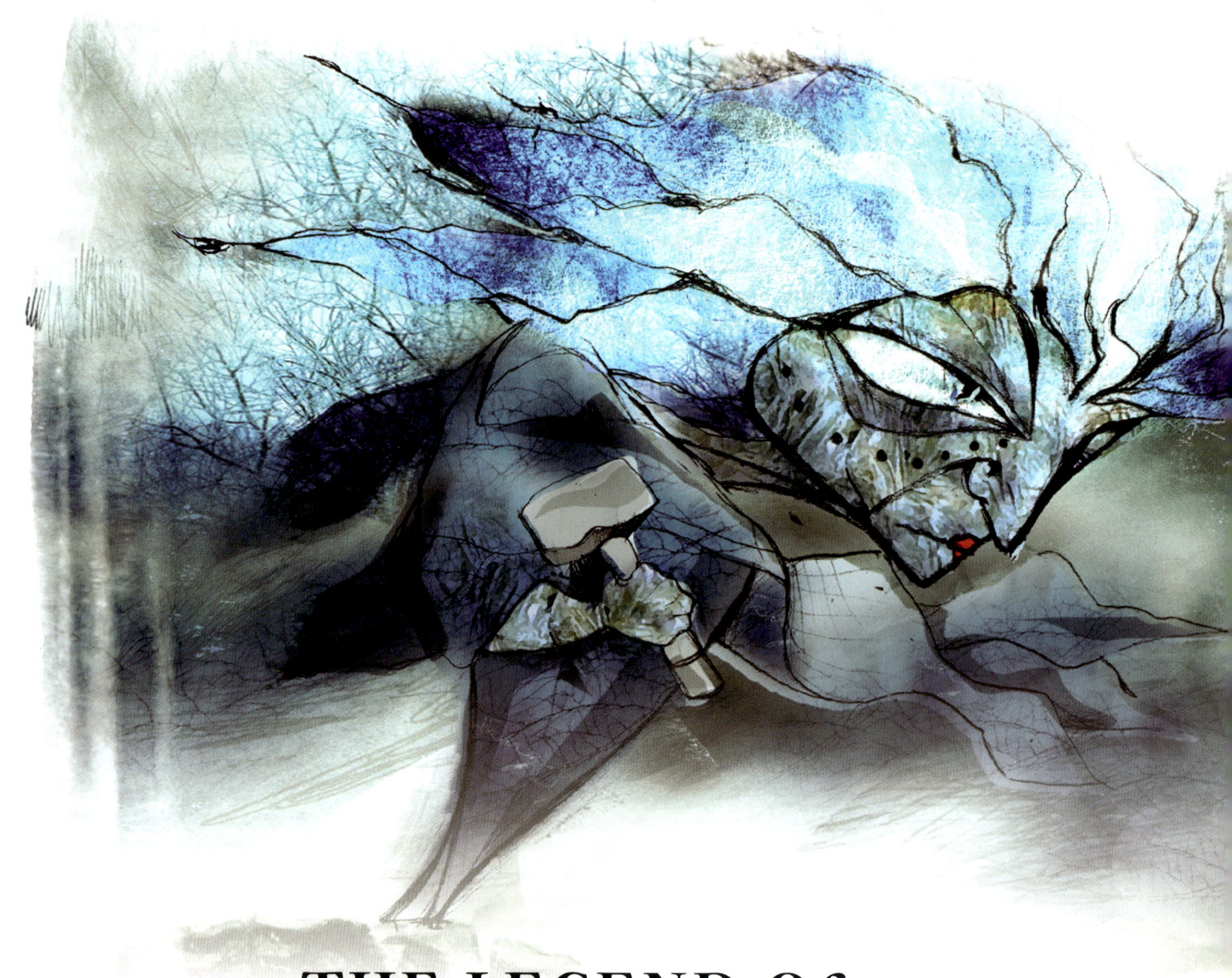

THE LEGEND OF BEIRA AND BRIDE

In the wild days of February, one moment the sky is blue and the sun is shining, then the next the wind is set to blow you over and the snow is falling. You may think that there is some sort of battle of the elements going on. Well, you'd be right! And here is the story behind the feud.

Long, long, long ago at the beginning of time, Nine Maidens lived at the bottom of the ocean. There they pushed with all their might at a great millstone, and earth came forth. Each woman wore a creel upon her back and these they filled with clods of clay. Then they set off around the world, creating the Earth as we now know it.

The oldest and ugliest of all the maidens was called Beira. She was the hag, the 'cailleach', the Goddess of Winter. Her skin was dull grey and wrinkled like a walnut. Her hair was as white as a hard frost and she only had one eye, but it had the vision of a hawk's. Her teeth were only a few stumpy, rusted pegs, and around her shoulders she wore a knitted shawl. In her hands she carried a hammer and a hazel switch, which she used to batter down any signs of growth or spring. No buds would flourish with Beira around, since her mission was to halt the coming of spring.

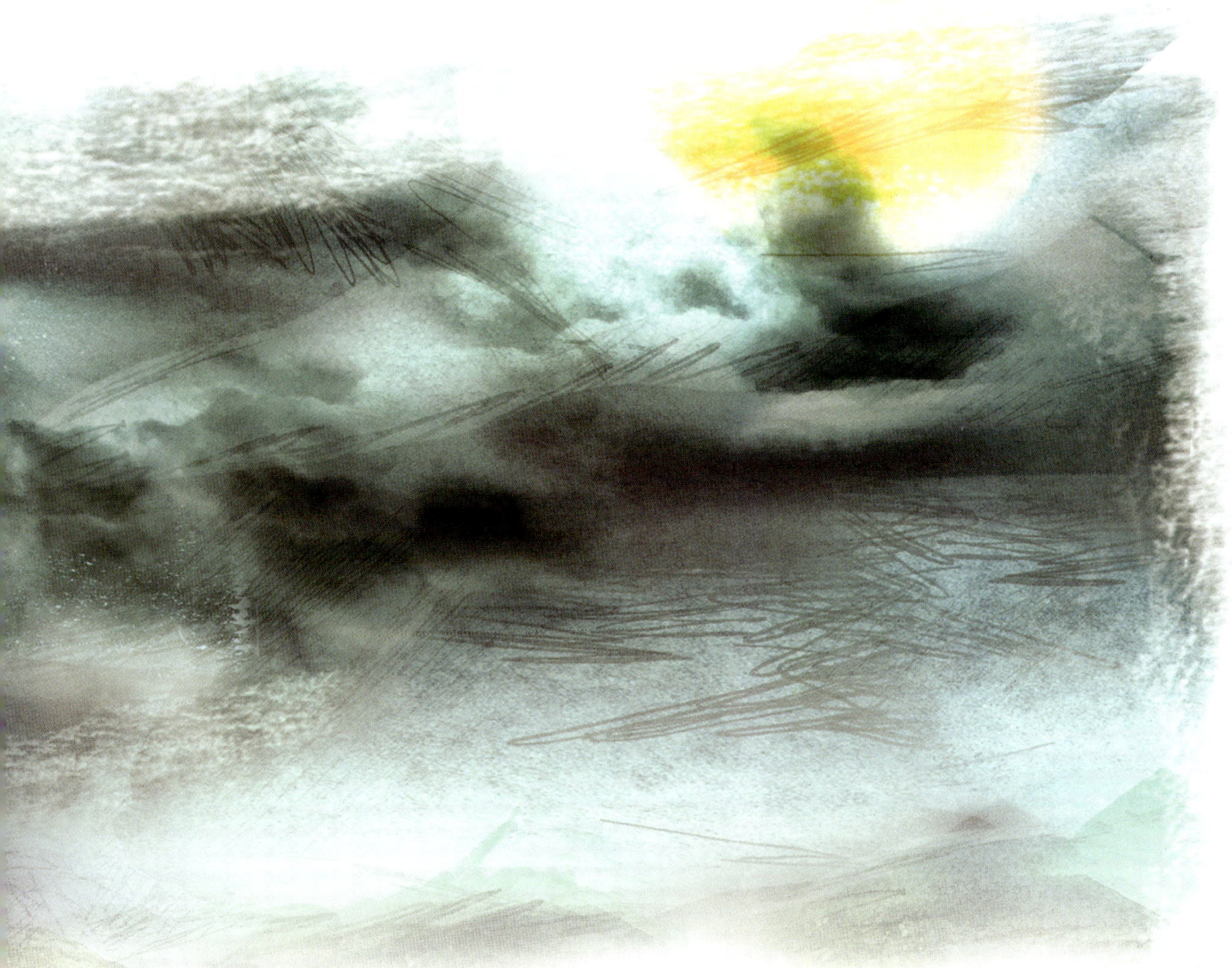

As her tired old bones carried her northwards, Beira became the sculptor of Scotland's landscape. Lumps of turf fell from her creel into the cold sea, and these made the mountains of Scotland. Wherever she crashed her heavy hammer into the earth, holes filled with water and the lochs of Scotland were formed.

For her home Beira chose the highest mountain in the land, Ben Nevis, and inside this mountain she lived with all her slaves and hags to look after her. But Beira felt old, sad, cold and alone.

One slave was called Nessa, and at sunset her job was to always cover up the water spring which Beira liked to use. If it was not covered, then the water flowed down the side of the mountain all night long, which displeased Beira. One night Nessa forgot her duty and in a panic she chased the water down the side of the mountain at sunset. A furious Beira saw her, and changed Nessa into water, crying, "Aye lassie, you'll run now and you'll run for evermore!"

This river of water then formed a loch that has become known as Loch Ness. If you listen by its banks on still summer nights, folk say you can hear the sad lament of Nessa's song. She is forever trapped in the waters of the loch.

When Beira wanted to do her washing she stepped out into the sea on the west coast, and there she stirred up the waters, making a washtub of swirling foam. This is known today as the Corryvrecken Whirlpool. She then threw her clean, white shawls over the mountaintops of Scotland to dry. To you and me these look like snow-covered peaks, but now you know what they truly are!

One day Beira chose a new slave, a beautiful young girl called Bride. Beira took a particular dislike to her. She demanded that Bride wash a dirty fleece and not return to her until it was spotless. Bride scrubbed it in the ice-cold stream until her hands were blue and sore, but still it would not come clean. Out of the woods came an old man, and with tears in her eyes she looked pleadingly at him.

"Why do you look so sad, lass?" he asked with a kindly smile.

"I must wash this fleece for my mistress Beira, but it will not come clean no matter how hard I scrub."

"Ah! Let me try!" He took the fleece and shook it once, twice, three times, and then it was as white as new snow!

"I am Father Winter," he said, and then handed a bunch of snowdrops to Bride, saying, "Here, take these to your mistress and tell her that the green buds are growing in the green woods."

With great relief, Bride scampered back to Beira and proudly showed her the white fleece. But Beira's hawk eye was fixed on the snowdrops and she roared, "Where did you get those?"

Bride cheerfully gave her the message from Father Winter, but Beira grabbed the snowdrops, and crushed the little flowers under her foot.

She snatched her birch switch and hammer, then mounted her grey horse, shrieking that she must go and stop the advance of spring. She flew across the sky, with her hags riding on goats trotting on the grey clouds behind her.

Meanwhile, off the west coast of Scotland, there lived Angus Og, the God of Summer. He floated on the Isle of Summer where the land was green and bountiful. One morning he sought out his father, Dagda, urgently saying, "I have dreamt many nights now about a young woman who I know is my heart's love. I must find her, for her eyes are brimming with tears. I will leave today."

But Dagda replied, "No, you must not leave now, for the month is February, the month of the Wolf, and the weather may be wild. Stay, rest and wait until summer."

"My heart cannot wait!" exclaimed Angus. "I will go to the God of August and ask for three summer days to be carried into the beginning of February so that I may travel immediately."

And so it was that his wish was granted. As Angus set off on his search, the seas flattened, the wind calmed and the sun began to shine. These first three days of February are still known as 'The Days of Bride', and the weather on these days is expected to be mild and fair.

He searched for his love all over the land and at last he found Bride at Ben Nevis. When she saw him she said, "I have seen your face in my dreams and at last you have come!" Bride shed tears of joy, and where they landed on the earth, violets sprang forth, bearing the same blue colour as her eyes.

So Angus took her by the hand and led her to the green woods, saying, "Now we shall be wed and you shall be the Goddess of Spring." As they walked, crocuses and snowdrops sprang forth in their wake. A frozen stream flowed once more with one touch of Bride's gentle hand.

In the heart of the woods they were greeted by the Fairy Queen. She changed

Bride's rags into a beautiful white and silver gown with one wave of her silver wand. Angus picked Bride a posy of flowers and all the birds of the air began to sing, heralding the arrival of spring. During the wedding the Linnet sang a glorious song and so became known as the 'Bird of Bride'. The Oyster-catcher looked on, wearing his smart black and white suit, and to this day is known as the 'Page of Bride'. Angus then took his bride to the Summer Isle and said, "Wait here, I must go and do battle with Beira."

Meanwhile, Beira and her hags smashed buds, crushed blossoms and breathed their ice-cold breath all over the land. As she rode forth, Beira summoned her ally, the fierce North Wind to ride with her, and dark grey storm clouds tumbled from her horse's hooves.

Angus, with his warm breeze and sunshine, still does battle with Beira's frosty army over the skies all through February and March. Around the 22nd of March, Beira makes a last attempt at destruction, with the high spring tides. But she will surely lose. Tired, sad and lonely, she then returns to the Summer Isle and there takes her rest beside the pool of Eternal Youth. She sips from the waters and sleeps a deep restful sleep. But she will awaken at Samhain, often now called Halloween, and then return once more to rule as the Goddess of Winter.

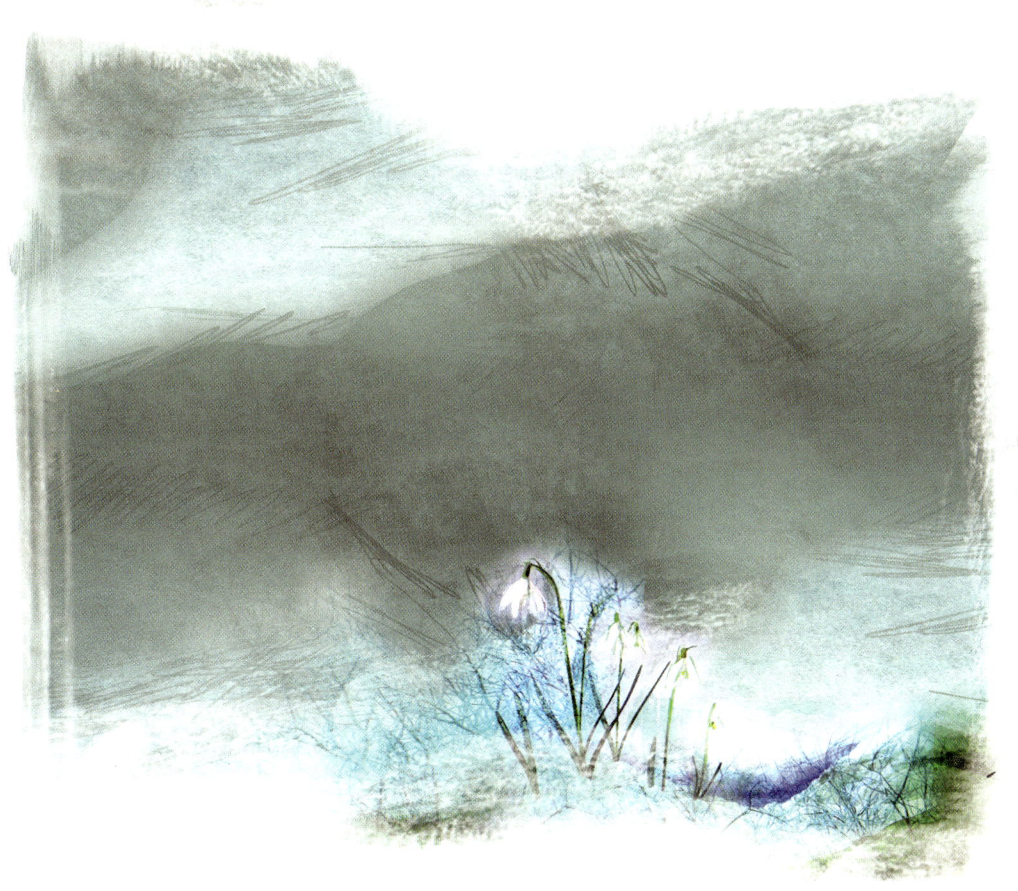

Follow-on Activity 1

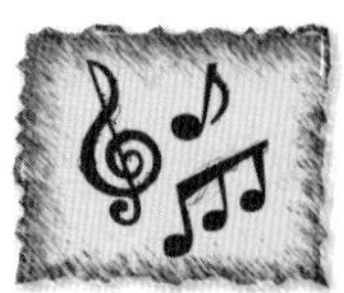

Story Soundscape

This story takes us to a variety of landscapes with many different characters. These all lend themselves to creating a 'Story Soundscape'. The aim of this activity is to create a version of the story with sound effects (although not necessarily formal music; don't be afraid of this exercise if you cannot play an instrument).
A soundscape may be done separately, or may accompany a telling of the story.

Aims

- To engage particularly with children who have a strong musicality but are verbally quiet. This exercise allows them to express ideas, thoughts and feelings and to participate fully in the story without having to talk.
- To encourage children to consider the moods and emotions in the story
- To give children the freedom to explore and enjoy playing with sounds and rhythms
- To encourage sensitivity to the spoken word, and the auditory association and visual images which a story can evoke

Materials

Anything that the children suggest, or may be keen to improvise, including;

- Percussion and other instruments (e.g. rain-stick, shaker, drum, bells, thunder-maker, thumb piano, lyre)
- Everyday objects, such as plastic bottles, newspapers, pens and rulers
- Body percussion (drumming of hands or feet, clapping, etc.)
- Mouth music, and oral sound effects (hissing, whooshing, etc.)

Method

Ask the children to consider the main elements of the story (see 'Story Skeleton' at the beginning of this chapter):

- The characters: the Nine Maidens, Beira, Nessa, Bride, Father Winter, Angus Og, Dagda, the Fairy Queen, the North Wind
- The action: fast or slow, exciting or calm
- The settings: the sea, the sky, the mountains, the lochs
- The moods: the fury of battle, the joy of a wedding

Invite each child (or group of children) to pick an instrument and explore what sounds it can make. Then ask the children to show their instruments one at a time. (Except for the one being discussed, all instruments should be placed on the floor so they cannot be fiddled with.) Ask to hear what kind of sound each instrument makes, and what kind of emotion, mood or action it might suggest.

Discuss what sounds and instruments may be evocative for each part of the story. Each character may be assigned a particular instrument or refrain. For example, a drum roll might represent Beira whenever she appears.

Children who play a formal instrument may also join in. Some children not experienced with a formal instrument may enjoy playing a single chord or note either at dramatic moments, or as a cue.

You and the children may decide to have sound effects or music for parts of the story only. Or you may choose to render the whole story in sound, without accompanying words.

Select which parts of the story should have sound effects or music, and map them out (coloured pens are useful to indicate different groups of instruments). Agree on how much the children should play and at what volume and tempo.

A conductor and a storyteller need to be appointed.

Ensure everybody has their instruments ready, and knows their entry points.

It works well for space to be left between the speaking and the ‘sounds’, rather than have the teller competing with the music.

The soundscape can be recorded and then listened to again.

If you have chosen to create a soundscape without any spoken words, it can be interesting to record this and then play it to children who didn’t hear the story being told, and ask them to guess what it was about.

Follow-on Activity 2

Make a Creation Myth

The story of Beira explains the landscape of Scotland and how it came to be. Beira created the mountains, the Corryvreckan Whirlpool and Loch Ness. Perhaps Beira also travelled widely and was responsible for creating things all over the world!

This exercise allows children to compose a creation myth of their own. Most cultures have such stories, explaining where things come from and why they look the way they do. Children show enthusiasm for this task, and often come up with humorous or thought-provoking possibilities. There is no right or wrong in story-making!

Aims

- To stimulate the imagination and a sense of meaning
- To promote working with others and sharing ideas
- To encourage a sense of cause and effect, conveyed within a structured story
- To enhance storytelling skills

Materials

Any visual prompts which may give children ideas for their own creation myth, such as postcards or pictures of

- Iconic Scottish symbols (haggis, thistle, highland cow, kippers, bagpipes) and landmarks (Arthur's Seat, the Firth of Forth, Ailsa Craig)
- Local landmarks
- World-famous landmarks

Method

Invite the children to make up a story titled "How Beira Created . . . ".
The story need only be two minutes long.
Children may work individually, in pairs, or in small groups.
Organise the children to tell their stories to the rest of the group.

This activity can be done as an oral exercise at first, and then be developed into a written format.

Follow-on Activity 3

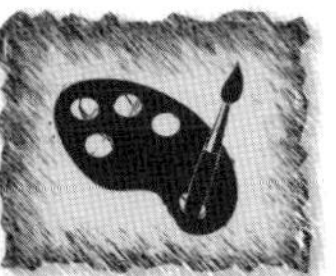

Woven Snowflake

In this story, Beira, Goddess of Winter, loves the cold, the North Wind and snow. On different days, the children can be asked "Who is winning the battle of the seasons today? Beira or Angus?"

A calendar can be used to track the dates mentioned in the story.
Weaving snowflakes from wool or ribbon, and hanging them in the window, allows you to decorate the room with a flavour of winter that Beira would enjoy!

Aims

- To give children a reflective, quiet task, during which they can be asked to think about the value of all the seasons, and the inevitable progress of time
- To encourage children to notice and observe the weather and seasons
- To develop hand and eye coordination

Materials

- Wooden craft sticks
- Wool or other type of yarn
- Optional extras or variations: fluffy wool, sparkling cords, silver or white ribbon
- Glue

Method

Glue the craft sticks together, criss-crossing them in the middle to form a star. Leave to dry.

Tie one end of the yarn around one stick in the centre of the 'stick star'. Take the yarn over the next stick. Pull behind and then weave the yarn around the front of the next stick. Keep the yarn tight whilst going 'over and under' the sticks, round in a circle. Repeat until all the sticks are nearly covered.

To finish, glue the end of the yarn to a stick. Make a loop, and attach to a longer length of yarn. Hang in the window on display.

If the snowflake is woven more loosely, light can shine through the yarn. Sparkling cords, fluffy wool, or even very fine silver or white ribbon can change the effect. Add little dabs of glitter glue all over the finished snowflake for extra sparkle.

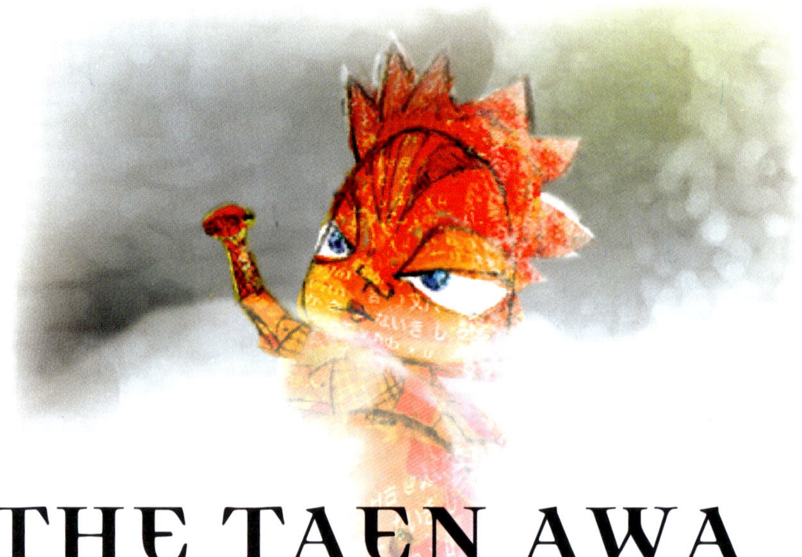

THE TAEN AWA

Introduction

Stage Primary 2 (age 6) upwards

Synopsis
This story echoes the old belief that a human baby could be taken away by the fairies and a 'bad' fairy left in its place, especially on the first day of May. In 'The Taen Awa', the mother doesn't notice the change, although she is distressed by the baby's constant and uncharacteristic crying.
The bad fairy reveals itself to the postman, who works out what must be done to retrieve the human baby. The mother follows his instructions and the family is restored.

Background
This Scottish tale is a great story to tell on or around May Day, and despite its discomfiting premise, tends to be popular.

Children can join in with the crying of the baby, and enjoy suggesting ways to soothe an infant. A baby doll may be used as a prop, which can then be passed around the listeners.

Suggested Themes

- The birth of a baby: the joys and challenges
- How appearances can be deceptive
- The usefulness of advice from someone who is wise
- The symbolic cleansing power of water
- The power of love
- Being given a second chance

Skeleton

1. Margaret and Malcolm marry and live on a croft.
2. They soon have a lovely boy, baby Malcolm, named after his father. Baby Malcolm is a calm baby, and rarely cries.
3. Malcolm asks Margaret to help him cut grass to make hay. It is the first day of May, when fairies are particularly active.
4. Margaret takes the baby out into the field and is surprised when he starts to cry.
5. Margaret tries everything she can think of to soothe him.
6. He cries until the sun sets, and begins again the next morning at sunrise.
7. He cries for days but no one, not even the doctor, can find anything wrong with him.
8. The postman visits, and suspecting that something strange is going on, offers to look after the baby while Margaret and Malcolm have a break.
9. Margaret and Malcolm go to the market in town while the postman minds the baby.
10. The baby reveals itself as a Taen Awa, a bad fairy. To the postman's amazement, it stops crying, leaps out of the cot, and holds its own mischievous ceilidh.
11. When Margaret and Malcolm return, the postman tells Margaret that her baby has been taken away by the fairies, to the Fairy Hill. She must throw the bad fairy into the waterfall. Then her baby will be returned to her.
12. Margaret does as the postman says, and the bad fairy shouts and curses the postman.
13. Margaret rushes home and finds baby Malcolm safe in his cradle.

THE TAEN AWA

In the month of May the fairies are out and about, so you had better watch out! On the first day of the month, May Day, they leave their winter dwellings and flit to their summer homes. But while they are among humankind they take the chance to cause mischief.

Now some fairies are just a little mischievous, and some are rather naughty. But a few are downright bad! The mischievous ones might move your mum's car keys. The naughty ones might hide your granny's glasses, but the bad ones . . . well, look out! Their favourite trick is to steal a human baby and put a bad fairy in its place!

In the north-west Highlands a young man called Malcolm lived on a croft, as his parents had before him. He courted Margaret, a teacher in the village school, and asked her to marry him. After being wed she gave up work to help Malcolm on the farm. A year later, when Margaret announced that she was to have a baby, Malcolm said she had made him the happiest man in the world! Margaret had a sweet baby boy and named him Malcolm, just like his daddy. He was so calm, so placid, that he almost never cried.

One fine May Day, Malcolm decided to cut some grass in order to have some food for the cow later in the year. The weather was fine and dry – the best time for cutting. But he didn't think he could manage it all by himself. So Margaret offered to help.

"What about baby Malcolm?" asked his daddy.

"He'll be no trouble," replied Margaret. "I'll take him with us in his wooden crib and he'll be quite happy." So she took him out to the field and placed him on a hillock in the middle of the field.

"I can keep an eye on him there," she said. Then they picked up their scythes and began to cut the grass.

It wasn't long before baby Malcolm began to grizzle and whine and cry. This was unusual for the wee lad, and so Margaret was puzzled. She immediately picked him up, and began to try all the ways to settle a crying baby.

She rubbed his back, in case he had wind. But he cried and cried.

She gave him a drink of milk, but he spat it out and kept on crying.

She checked his nappy, but it was dry and he kept on crying.

She sang his favourite song, 'Ally Bally Bee', but he kept on crying.

She checked all over his body for a rash or bee sting, but she could see no marks and he kept on crying.

At last she said to Malcolm, "I shall take him home and try to settle him there." But even at home Malcolm kept on crying. In fact, he cried until the moment the sun sank behind the hills. Finally, Margaret was able to get some peace.

But as soon as the sun rose again the next morning, baby Malcolm began to cry. He went on and on, all day long. Margaret was beside herself, and Malcolm suggested that they visit the doctor. So they did.

The doctor listened to baby Malcolm's chest, looked inside his ears, felt his tummy, and then announced that he could find nothing wrong.

Baby Malcolm cried the whole day, but when the sun sank behind the hills he stopped. And when the sun rose again the next morning he started once more.

That day there came a knock at the door. It was the postman. He had known Margaret and Malcolm all their lives, and since they lived outside the village, he was their most frequent visitor. The postman could see that Margaret looked very tired and drawn. "What's wrong, lass?" he asked.

"Oh, Postie! You have no idea! It's baby Malcolm! He has cried non-stop for days. We don't know what's wrong with him," said Margaret.

"Well now," said the postman, "I've learnt a bit about bairns over the years, so I'll have a look at him if you like."

The postman looked at baby Malcolm and immediately thought that he seemed a little bit strange. His eyes seemed to have an extra sparkle, and his skin looked old and leathery. Then the postman had an idea.

"Look here," he said to Margaret, "I've come to tell you that there is a market in town today, so why don't you and Malcolm take yourselves off and have a break. I'll look after the wee lad."

"Oh, Postie, I couldn't leave you here with a crying baby," said Margaret. "It would drive you mad!"

"I'll be fine," insisted the postman, and so with a little more persuasion, Margaret and Malcolm brought out the horse and cart and headed off to the market.

Baby Malcolm lay in his crib, grizzling away to himself. However, as soon as the sound of horses' hooves was out of earshot, the baby sat up and stopped crying.

He leapt out of his crib and announced proudly, "Now, Postie, we're goin' tae hae oorsels a ceilidh! Ye'll niver hae heard better music in your life."

Then he ran across the room, his nappy dangling between his legs, and headed for the cabinet.

"This is whaur the whisky is!" he yelled excitedly. He pulled on the door, but it was locked.

He put a finger into his mouth and gave it a good suck. Then he pushed his finger into the lock, and as if by magic, it opened. He took out a whisky bottle and two glasses, and poured out two large drams. Passing one to the postman, he cried, "Slainte! Guid health!" and gulped down the whisky. The postman's eyes were nearly popping out of his head; he couldn't believe what he was seeing.

The peculiar baby went outside and returned with a stalk of straw. He then stuck the poker into the fire. When the poker was hot, he burned tiny holes into the stalk, making it into a straw whistle. Then he started to play, and danced all around the room, full of the joy of his own music.

When the sound of approaching hooves could be heard, the baby hitched up his nappy, ran across to the fire and threw his whistle onto the flames. When Margaret and Malcolm walked through the door, he was back lying in his crib, howling to the rafters.

"Oh, my wee bairn!" exclaimed Margaret, rushing to the crib. "He's no better!" she said in despair. "Oh, Postie, has he been greeting the whole time? You must have a headache."

"I can't begin to tell you what's been goin' on here. I need to talk to you in private, straight away!" whispered the postman. They stepped outside together.

"That's no baby in there! It is a bad fairy and your own wee Malcolm has been taken away to the Fairy Hill. Now, there is only one way to get him back and you have to trust me on this. Did you buy a new blanket today?" Margaret nodded.

"Well," he continued, "take the blanket and wrap the fairy firmly within. Be sure that its hands are tucked away securely, or it may clutch you and carry you to your doom. Then you must take it to the head o' the glen, to the top of the waterfall. Throw the fairy into the rushing water, and when you come home, your own baby Malcolm will have been returned."

"Oh, my goodness," exclaimed Margaret. "Are you sure?"

"Margaret, you've known me all your life. And this way of dealing with a Taen Awa was told to me by my own granny, who was wise in the ways of fairies. Believe me, this is the only way!"

Margaret was not so sure, but did as she was told. She wrapped up the leathery-faced sprite and made her way to the top of the waterfall. She looked down at the sharp rocks and at the rushing water, deafened by its thundering music. She remembered the postman's words, and, drawing on all her resolve, threw the bundle down, down into the waterfall.

As it hit the pool of water far below, the fairy sat up in the water. He shook his fist, and shouted, "Had I known Postie would tell on me, then I would niver hae given him whisky or my guid music!" With that, he was washed away by the current.

Margaret hurried home as quickly as she could, anxious about what she might find. She ran to the crib, and there, gurgling happily, lay her own baby Malcolm.

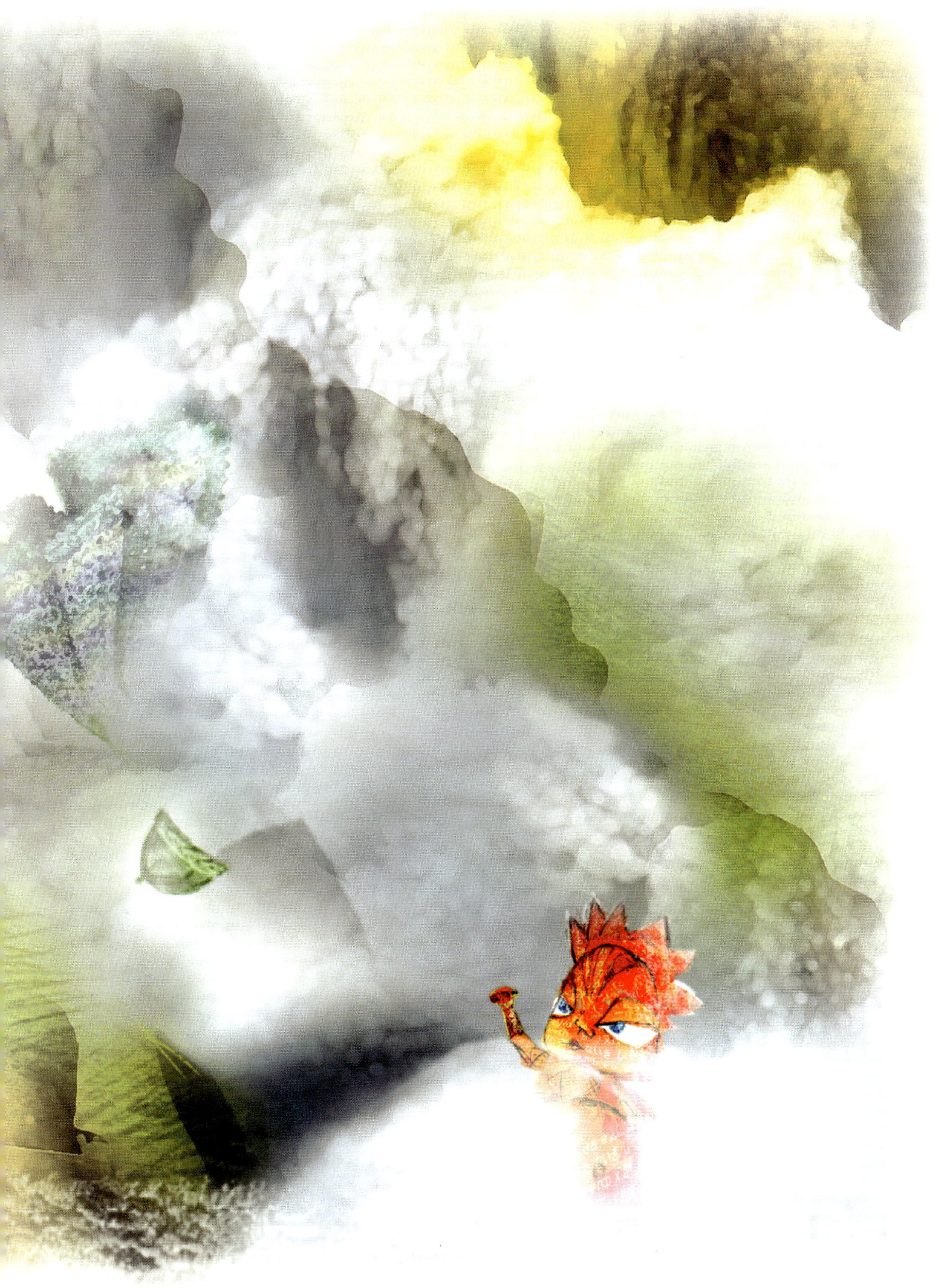

Follow-on Activity 1

Baby Care

During this story, we are told that baby Malcolm was crying and seemed upset. Margaret tried to comfort him.

Babies generally cry when there is something wrong, but what can we do to make them feel better?

In this exercise, the children are asked to consider a baby's needs for care and comfort, and how this is not so different from their own needs.

A baby doll can be a useful aid.

Aims

- To encourage children to think about a baby's needs
- To highlight that babies' needs are not so different from ours
- To develop empathy and patience

Materials

- Just the group!
- Optionally, a baby doll

Method

This exercise may be done during the story, at a point when baby Malcolm is crying inconsolably, or else after it.

Alternatively, the first part of the exercise may be done during the story, and the second part afterwards.

Working in pairs, ask the children to think of three or more ways to soothe a crying baby. Collect suggestions from the group. For example:

1. Rubbing the baby's back and gently patting it, in case wind is causing discomfort
2. Offering some milk
3. Singing a lullaby
4. Picking the baby up and giving him or her a cuddle
5. Distracting the baby with a soft toy
6. Taking the baby for a walk in the pram

Next, instead of thinking about babies, direct the children to thinking about themselves.

When they are upset are there ways that they can be comforted?
Ask them to think of three or more ways that someone could use to help them to feel better. Collect suggestions from the group. For example:

1. Asking what is wrong, then listening with understanding
2. Offering a reassuring hug or cuddle
3. Offering a drink or a snack
4. Reading, or telling, a story
5. Playing a favourite game together
6. Going for a walk or bicycle ride together

The conclusion is that the needs of babies are not so different from ours. What is different, however, is that babies cannot talk, and so need extra gentleness, patience and understanding.

Follow-on Activity 2

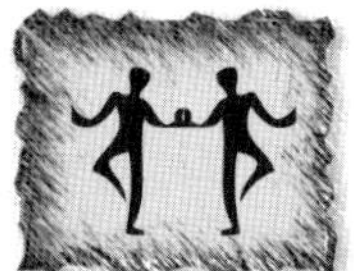

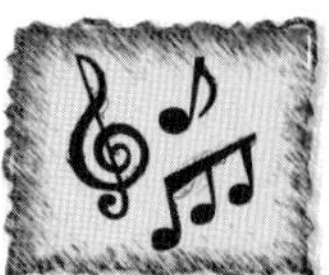

Make a Waterfall

In this story the bad fairy is dropped into a roaring waterfall by Margaret.

This group exercise echoes the sound of the waterfall as Margaret hurries towards the hilltop, a distant murmur growing to a thunderous roar. Then, as she turns for home, the sound of the cascading water recedes and fades away to silence.

The children, using their hands and feet, build the sound of the waterfall steadily, layer by layer, to a crescendo. Then the sound gradually diminishes to nothing as the children reverse their orchestration.

This activity requires concentration, with the children following the actions of the leader in turn, timing their entry points, and expressing each layer of sound in a steady, rhythmic way. To accomplish all this, the children must listen to each other, observe and cooperate.

It's an enjoyable activity, leading to a feeling of shared satisfaction as the sound of the waterfall builds, peaks and ebbs in a coordinated fashion.

Aims
- To build concentration
- To encourage the group to think about working in a cohesive way
- To promote observation skills

Materials
- Just the group, using their hands and feet

Method
Arrange the children so that they are seated on chairs, in a circle.

Explain that they are going to create the sound of the waterfall in the story, growing louder and then fading as Margaret approaches and then turns home.

Nominate one person (the practitioner in the first run-through) to act as leader, or conductor.

There will be four stages in this orchestration (rather like a symphony, with four movements). The different sounds in each stage come from a different action. Allow about a minute for each stage.

1. Rubbing hands
2. Clicking fingers
3. Slapping thighs
4. Slapping thighs and stamping feet

The leader begins by doing the first action (with its accompanying sound) in a steady, rhythmic way.

After a few seconds, the person on the leader's right joins in.

After a few more seconds, the leader cues the next person in the circle, who joins in.

This continues around the circle until the whole group is doing the same action and making the same sound.

The leader then changes to the next action and accompanying sound, but the rest of the group must continue making the previous sound until it is their turn to change.

The 'waterfall symphony' should gradually build, layer by layer, to a peak, when all in the circle are slapping their thighs and stamping their feet.

Then, keep going, but reversing the stages, until the only the sound of rubbing hands is heard.

On the very last round, the leader stops rubbing, and then cues the person on the right to stop, and so on, until all is silence.

Follow-on Activity 3

Story Maps

In this activity, the children are asked to make an illustrated 'topographical' map of the story, showing places, characters and actions. It can be rather like a 'treasure map', or, say, a map of Narnia, but with the addition of stick figures or symbols representing what happens in different locations.

Story maps are an alternative to a cartoon strip or a storyboard (a series of drawings showing the order of events in a story). Like a storyboard, a story map is mostly pictorial, but it illustrates the 'journey' of a story across an imagined landscape as well as through time.

Creating a map can help children to identify the basic elements and the chronology of a story, breaking down the 'who', 'where', 'why', 'when' and 'what' of the narrative. Making a story map can be very useful in helping children to learn, analyse or write a story.

It can also be a bridge between a story as spoken, a story as imagined in the 'mind's eye', and a story as depicted in words or drawn images.

Aims

- To help children to picture the story and understand the sequence of events
- To help children learn the story

Materials

- Plain A4 or A3 paper
- Alternatively, an outline or skeleton map can be designed, copied, and given to each child to fill in or embellish
- Coloured pens or pencils

Method

Explain the concept of a story map to the children.

The practitioner can give the children a template designed in advance, or they can develop their own style of map.

Emphasise that this activity doesn't require artistic skill, since stick people, words and symbols can be used, and the map may be diagrammatic rather than 'realistic'. Encourage the children to be creative in how they depict the story on paper, explaining that each map is likely to look different, despite being inspired by the same tale.

Ask the children, in planning their maps, to consider the 'where', 'when', 'who', 'what' and 'why' of the story. Since a map is being drawn, it's probably best to consider 'where' first (for location), then 'when' (for chronology), associated with 'who' (characters), 'what' (what happens to them), and 'why' (motives and feelings behind their actions).

- 'Where': the different locations (farmhouse, field, doctor's surgery, road to town, market, waterfall)
- 'When': arrows or numbers can show the order of action
- 'Who': the characters (Margaret and Malcolm, baby Malcolm, the bad fairy, the doctor, the postman), and (for older children) any details about them (feelings, personality traits, motives) which might be represented symbolically (e.g. a heart for Margaret, a hat or a scythe for Malcolm, a cradle or bottle for baby Malcolm, with tears added for 'crying Malcolm', a stethoscope, bag or red cross for the doctor, an envelope for the postman, a straw whistle for the bad fairy). More simply, initials or a stick figure might be used to show characters at the relevant locations.
- 'What': what is happening to whom (e.g. baby Malcolm being left during the grass-cutting might be represented by a cradle on top of a mound, in the middle of a field)
- 'Why': the reasons and emotions behind the characters' actions might be difficult to render visually (such as when Margaret, worried, takes 'baby Malcolm' to the doctor), but (particularly for older children) it can be worth asking the children to consider how the characters are feeling as the story progresses (and as they move through the story map). Question marks or exclamation marks can be useful. For instance, Margaret's anxiety at the doctor's might be represented by '???', and the postman's reaction to the jigging fairy might be '??!!!'!

FINN McCOOL AND THE YOUNG HERO'S CHILDREN

Introduction

Stage Primary 4 (age 8) upwards

Synopsis
Finn McCool, the great Ulster warrior, is helped by a strange band of men and women, each with a specific skill. Together they rescue three children who have been snatched away from their parents by a giant. Each of their skills is vital to the rescue.

Background
There are many tales of Finn, but this is one of the best. It gives an introduction to the world of Finn and the Fianna. It is a great story for building a sense of community in a group or class. It can be particularly useful in preparing for transition to high school.

A long story, it can be told in sections.

Suggested Themes
- The value of working as a team
- Everyone has something to contribute
- Challenges can be overcome by using our wits
- The power of love and loyalty
- Good will conquer evil

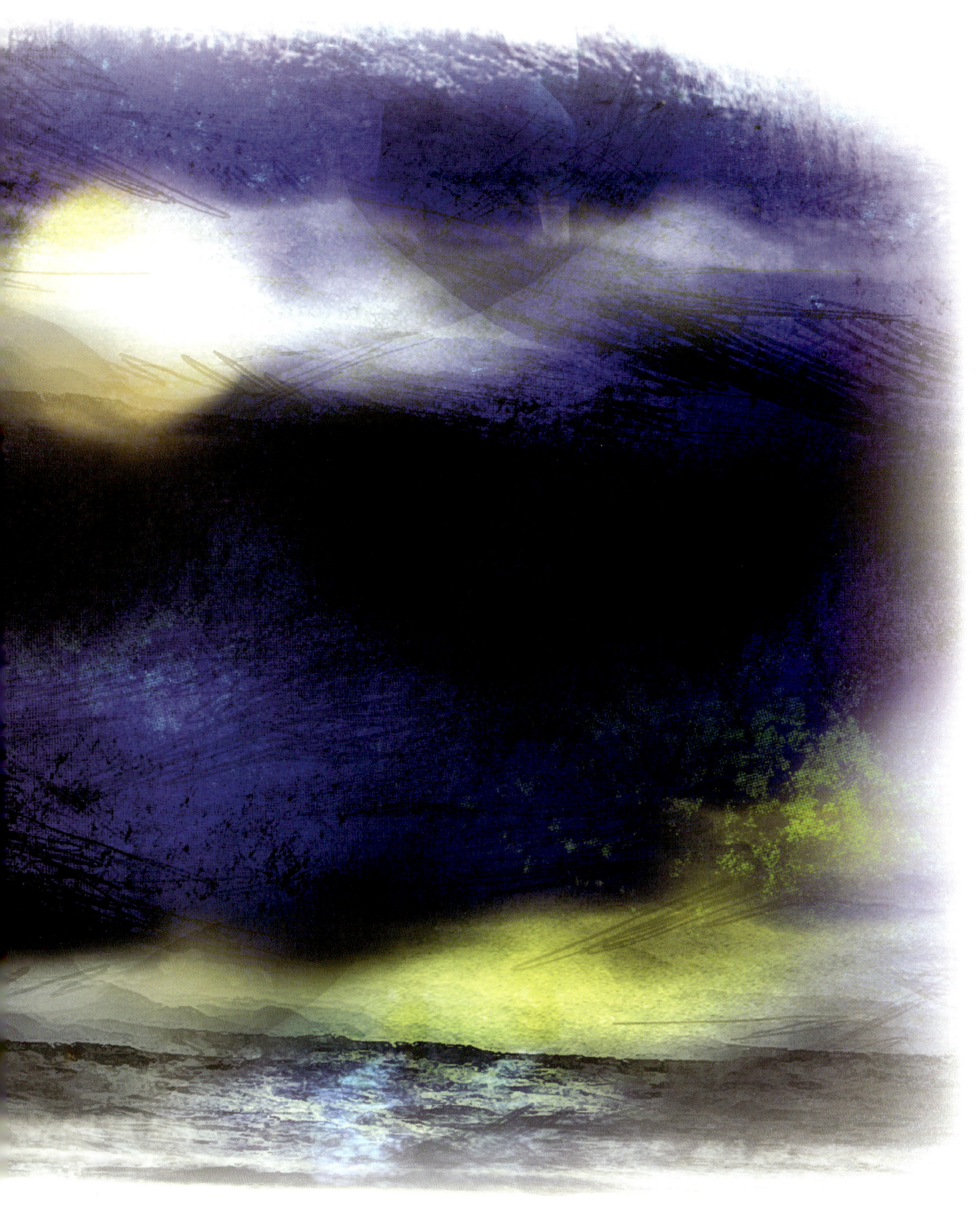

Skeleton

1. Finn is about to enjoy a feast on the beach with the Fianna.
2. A stranger (the Young Hero) arrives, arousing suspicion, for no one knows if he is friend or foe.
3. The stranger says that Finn is the only person who can help him, and then mysteriously disappears back out to sea.
4. Finn leaves the Fianna to their feast, and goes in search of the Young Hero.
5. He comes across a motley group, who offer assistance.
6. Finn asks what they are best at in the world, and they each describe their special skill. Finn gladly accepts the services of the Shipwright, the Tracker, the Climber, the Gripper, the Thief, the Listener and the Marksman.
7. Finn and the Helpers travel together in a new boat built by the Shipwright.
8. Led by the Tracker, they find the Young Hero.
9. The Young Hero explains that he has had two newborn sons snatched by a giant, and his wife is about to bear a third child.
10. The third child is born. He is suddenly snatched by the Giant reaching down through the chimney. The Gripper saves the child by ripping off the Giant's arm.
11. The Giant, however, suddenly reaches in with his other hand and steals the baby.
12. Finn promises to bring the child safely home.
13. The Tracker guides them across the sea to the Giant's island tower.
14. The Climber peers into the top of the tower and sees the Giant sleeping with the baby in his hand, and two small boys playing nearby. There is also a fierce mother Wolfhound suckling two pups.
15. The Climber carries the Thief up the tower, from where they rescue the children and take the pups.
16. Finn and the Helpers row desperately towards the Young Hero's home.
17. The Listener hears the furious Giant awakening, and orders the Wolfhound to pursue the ship. The Wolfhound, breathing fire, obeys.
18. Fearing that they would all be burnt alive, Finn throws one of the pups into the sea.
19. The mother chooses to rescue her pup from drowning, and abandoning the chase, swims with it back to the tower.

20. The Listener hears the Giant setting out himself after the Wolfhound refuses to leave her pup.
21. The Giant stretches out his hand to crush the boat, and Finn feels despair.
22. Despite his terror at their predicament, Finn remembers to press on his 'Tooth of Knowledge' (which since boyhood has provided him with solutions).
23. Finn tells the Marksman to shoot an arrow at the Giant's weak spot, a mole on his hand. The Giant is killed.
24. Finn and the Helpers fetch the Wolfhound and her pup.
25. They return the children to the Young Hero and his wife.
26. Finn is rewarded with a pup and names him Bran.

Finn McCool and the Young Hero's Children

Have you heard tell of the mighty Finn McCool? Some say that his name must be mentioned at least once every day, or the world will end. So if you are reading this aloud, you may have just saved the world!

Finn was a hero in the ancient lands of Alba, now known as Scotland, and of Erin, or Ireland. He had a band of faithful followers called 'the Fianna'. They were warriors, but skilled in the ways of peace as well as war. To join the Fianna they had to pass many tests of skill. They had to be able to run through a forest without breaking a twig, recite a great long ballad by heart, and defend themselves in a deep pit against a dozen sharp spears. They had to be great hunters, using wolfhounds to chase down the deer, boar and game birds that filled the forests in those bygone days. All the Fianna swore allegiance to the High King of Ireland, who sat on his throne at Tara, but it was Finn McCool who led them.

There are many tales of Finn and here is one of my favourites . . ..

On the heathery hillsides of Argyll, in the west of Scotland, Finn and his men had spent a fine day hunting. They were roasting a wild boar over an open fire on the beach, their energy spent, their bellies empty. Goll MacMorna, who had only one eye (yet he could see like a falcon), looked out to sea, and there on the horizon he saw a black speck. He cried, "We have company!" and in time the others could see a splendid ship headed for the shingle. As the boat neared the shore, a Young Hero with a gold band around his neck and a red silk cloak sprang from the prow and waded ashore. Squinting against the light, he peered at the men of the Fianna. His eyes fell on Finn and he asked, "Are you Finn McCool?"

"I am," said Finn.

The Young Hero's face relaxed as he proclaimed, "You are the only man on this wide earth who can help, and you must come with me!"

"But I am just about to feast," grumbled Finn.

"I put a 'geise' on you that you will never again eat, you will never again drink, and you will never again sleep, until you come to my aid." Then the young man turned on his heel and strode back down the beach, waded out to his boat and soon disappeared over the horizon.

Finn turned to his men and said, "You know what this means. I must go."

"Don't go, Finn," they said. "It's a trap! Who does he think he is, talking that way to you, the great Finn!"

"I have no choice," said Finn, "For well I know the power of the 'geise' and I will after all have to eat, drink and sleep! You feast and soon I will return." His men tried to persuade him to take a companion but he refused, and left alone.

Finn walked along the beach until he came to some rocks where he found seated a strange assembly of people. They spoke in unison, saying, "Can we be of help to you, Finn McCool?"

Finn looked from one to the other and to each he posed the question, "Well, what can you do best in all the world?"

A big sturdy man stood up. He had a leather bag slung over his shoulder with all manner of tools sticking out of it. "I am the Shipwright," he said. "Do you see those alder trees over there by the river? With three blows of my axe I could fell one and fashion you the finest ship you have ever set eyes upon."

"A shipwright? That's a very fine skill. Come with me!"

Next, Finn's eyes fixed upon a woman with a delicate aquiline nose and flared nostrils. She arose and answered, "Why, Finn, I am the Tracker. I can follow the path of a butterfly from the glen to the sea."

"Tracking! A most valuable skill," said Finn. "Come with me!"

A long lean woman stood up and stretched her gangly arms and legs. "I am the Climber," she said softly. "I could scramble to the very summit of a glass mountain!"

"Climbing is a most courageous skill," said Finn. "Come with me!"

A huge hulk of a man stood up and flexed his rippling biceps. "I am the Gripper. If I take hold of something my muscles lock and I will not let it go until it is mine."

"Ah, such physical strength is a handy skill", said Finn. "Come with me!"

Finn tipped a wink to a little wiry man hunched with age, his hands in perpetual motion, his fingers twining around themselves. "I am the Thief," he began. "My hands are so deft that I can take the eggs and the tail feathers from under a hen while she sits on her nest and she will not even know they are gone!"

"Well, thieving might be a useful skill," said Finn. "Come with me!"

Finn then turned to a woman whose delicate ears, which were fine as shells, sat out a little from her head. "I am the Listener," she whispered. "A snowflake may fall on the other side of the earth while I am asleep and I will hear it drop."

"Ah," said Finn, "Listening is the world's most precious skill. Come with me!"

Finally, a boy with a bow and arrow stood up eagerly as if not wanting to be forgotten. The young boy spoke proudly. "I am the Marksman. My aim is so true, I could shoot a single midge from the night sky."

"That is a vital skill," said Finn. "I will need all of your help. Come with me!"

The Shipwright was the first to go to work. He felled the alder trees and fashioned them into the finest ship they had ever seen. When all were on board, Finn stood at the prow with the Tracker by his side. She sniffed the air and studied the water, following the trail of the Young Hero. At last they came to an island green with hazel trees, where they beached their boat and went ashore. The Young Hero strode down the shingle to meet Finn and threw his arms wide in welcome. "You have come!" he cried.

"You did not leave me much choice," replied Finn. "After all, I must eat, drink and sleep!"

"There is no time for sleeping now," said the Young Hero. "But come and feast with me."

As they ate, the Young Hero told Finn his story. "Seven years ago I met a woman to whom I gave my heart's love. After a year of marriage we were blessed with the birth of a little baby boy. On the night he was born we thought we were the happiest souls on earth. But late that night, as my wife lay cherishing our newborn child, into the room came a huge, hairy blue hand, searching, searching for my child! The giant hand snatched my son from my wife's breast and I have never seen him since that night. We wept and we wailed and we thought we would never smile again, but a year later we discovered that we would be blessed with another child. On the night our second son was born he too was seized in the same way! Again, our hearts were broken. My wife is expecting another babe who will be born this very night. Finn, we cannot bear to lose another child. Only you can protect this precious little one."

Finn looked sorrowful, as he well knew the pain of a family torn by strife. He spoke with feeling. "I guarantee that your child will have my protection, and not only mine, but also the protection of my skilled companions who have come to my aid. Rest easy, for I will stay outside your wife's chamber and guard her throughout the night."

Finn sat outside, fighting sleep. To stay alert, he pushed his arm against the brass of the fireplace, burning his skin and waking himself up. Late that night, a little baby boy was born and placed gently in his mother's arms. Finn softly entered the room and saw the peaceful scene, with the proud mother nursing the contented babe at her breast.

Suddenly, a huge, hairy blue hand stretched down the chimney and began reaching for the little one. Finn cried out, "Gripper, Gripper! Come to my aid!"

The door was flung open and in strode the Gripper. He took hold of the giant wrist and held on determinedly as he was flung hither and thither. At last, with an almighty wrench, he tore the Giant's arm clean out of its socket, leaving a trail of blood and sinew. A huge wave of black blood gushed down the chimney and into the hall. The little baby lay still and safe in the limp hand of the Giant. But as everyone breathed a huge sigh of relief, into the room came another great hairy hand. It snatched the infant from the limp hand, and away!

Finn hung his head, unable to meet the young mother's grief-stricken eyes. "I give you my word," he promised, "I will not return to my own fireside until I have returned your child."

Without delay Finn and his helpers set sail. The Tracker stood at the prow of the boat with Finn and sniffed the air. As the sun set and night fell, she guided them to a tall tower which seemed to grow straight out of an island of rock. The roof shone silver in the moonlight. Finn's eyes roved around the boat until they fell upon the Climber. "This is a job for you," he said.

The Climber leapt cleanly from the boat and onto the wall of the tower. Up she crawled, like a spider. She was gone a very long time and when she dropped back into the boat she looked tired.

"Tell us what you saw," said Finn eagerly.

"Well, we have indeed found the Giant's lair, but the tower is a treacherous climb as the only entrance is in the roof and it is covered in slippery eel-skins. The Giant lies asleep with a silk sheet beneath him and a silk sheet over him. The place where his arm used to be is wrapped in a linen sheet soaked in blood and in the palm of his remaining hand lies the baby. In the same room there are two little

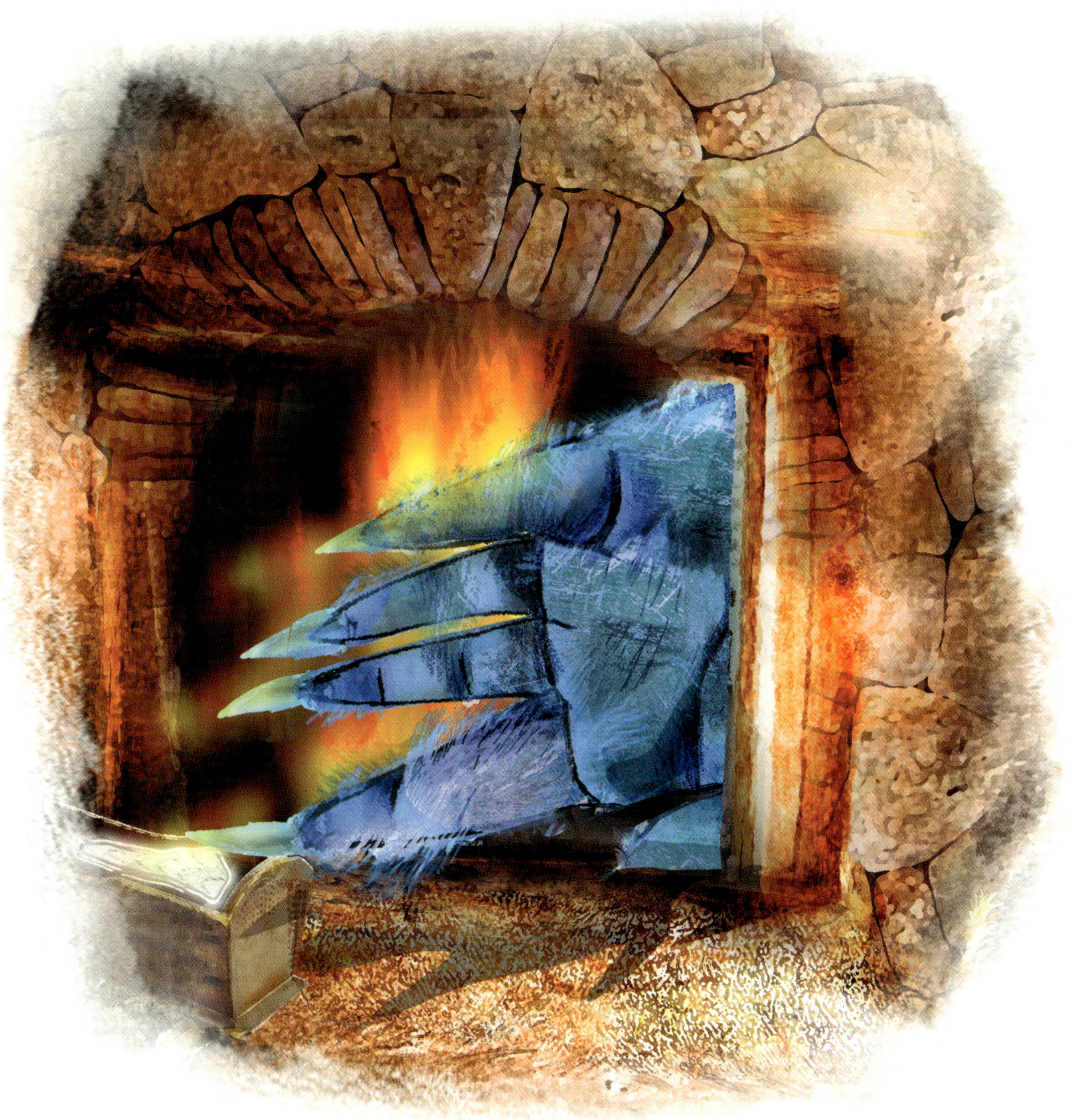

boys playing hurling with silver sticks and a golden ball. In the corner by the fire lies a huge wolfhound, suckling two pups.

Finn turned to the Thief. "This is a job for you," he said.

"But how am I to climb that tower?" asked the Thief.

"Why, with the help of the Climber, of course! Jump onto her back!" replied Finn.

So the Thief leapt onto the Climber's back and together they scaled the tall tower. The Thief sneaked into the Giant's bedchamber and took the baby, the two little boys, the hurley sticks, the golden ball, the two wolfhound pups (the dog herself was too fierce), the silk sheet from over the Giant, and, just to be cheeky, the silk sheet from beneath him.

As soon as the Climber and the Thief dropped down into the boat with all that they had gathered from the tower, Finn and his helpers began to row frantically towards the island of the Young Hero.

It was not long before the Listener said to Finn, "The Giant has woken up, for he was cold without the sheet over him. He is very angry, for we have taken from him everything he loves. He is sending the Wolfhound after us."

Looking to the horizon, they could see the huge Wolfhound with flames flaring from her nostrils. Finn's heart skipped a beat, for she was approaching swiftly, and he knew that when the flames reached the ship they would be burnt alive. But Finn was quick-thinking and he knew in an instant what to do.

And what do *you* think he would do?

He thought of the Wolfhound as a mother, and knew she would protect the life of her pup before trying to destroy the ship. So, as she drew near, Finn threw one of the pups overboard. Immediately the flames from the Wolfhound were extinguished as she swam towards her pup. She grabbed him gently by the scruff of his neck. Then she turned and swam back to the island of the Giant.

Finn and his helpers rowed with all their might, but it was not long before the Listener spoke up. "The Wolfhound has reached the Giant's tower. He is bellowing at her, telling her to come after us. But she is snarling at him and refusing to leave her pup. So now the Giant is rising up and coming after us himself!"

All of a sudden the sky darkened, and when they looked behind, they saw the Giant's bulk blocking out the light of the full moon. The Giant began stretching out his huge hairy hand towards the boat. Finn's heart sank as he saw that the ship would be crushed into tiny splinters by the Giant's mighty grip. What were they to do?

For a moment Finn's courage failed him and he thought that all was lost. But then he remembered a special gift given to him in boyhood: his 'Tooth of Knowledge'. Finn placed his thumb against his front tooth and in a flash he knew what to do. He saw that the Giant had one weak spot, a black mole in the palm of his remaining hand.

Finn sought the small boy, the Marksman, saying urgently, "You will only have one shot. You must not fail us. Aim for the mole in the centre of the Giant's palm."

"I will not fail," said the boy. Taking a deep breath, he drew back his bow, and waited until the Giant opened his hand to crush the ship. At the last moment, he let fly his golden arrow and it whirred through the air. It struck the Giant clean in the middle of his palm, piercing the black mole. The Giant gave a roar that split the sky and he fell backwards into the ocean. His form was so immense that a huge wave rose in his wake, tossing the ship high into the air.

Finn and his helpers held on tightly to the vessel and to their precious cargo, until the sea became calm. The moon vanished and on the horizon appeared the faint pink glow of dawn.

Finn saw the fatigue in the faces of his helpers. "I know you are weary," he said. "But our task is not yet complete, for we cannot leave a little wolfhound pup and his mother to perish alone in the Giant's tower. We must fetch them." And so they gathered the remains of their strength and rowed all the way back to the island of the Giant. As they rowed, the huge golden ball of the sun rose slowly out of the sea.

At the island, the Climber and the Thief scaled the tower again and returned with the Wolfhound and her pup. By now the Wolfhound was meek as a lamb, and yelped joyfully when reunited with her other pup.

The sun warm on their backs, the company rowed steadily until they reached the land of the Young Hero. Finn waded through the shallows to the shore, cradling the tiny baby in his arms, and with the two little boys riding on his shoulders. The Young Hero fell to his knees and wept in gratitude and relief. The family embraced, overjoyed at being reunited.

"Ask of me anything that you will, Finn McCool, and I will not refuse you," said the Young Hero.

Finn smiled warmly, thought for a moment and then gently said, "I ask only to choose one of these wolfhound pups."

Finn chose the brindled pup and named it Bran. And of Finn and Bran, his favourite hunting dog, there are many more tales to tell, but those are for another day.

Follow-on Activity 1

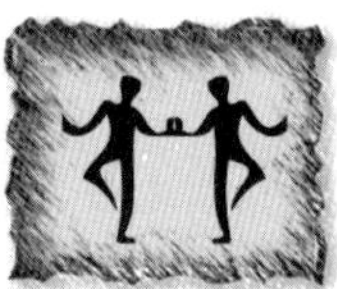

Arruchica

Remind the children that to be in the Fianna you had to be skilled. Members had to be fit both mentally and physically for battle, for negotiating peace, and for finding solutions to all kinds of dilemmas. Explain that this activity will test their level of fitness and ensure that they are ready for life's next challenge!

Tell the children that Finn McCool might have done this ritual of movement with the Fianna, his band of supporters. You might say that it is chanted in the language of the ancient Celts.

Part of the fun of this activity is to begin in a serious manner, and watch the children as they realise that the movements are becoming increasingly ridiculous, and that the ritual itself is a jest. Being able to laugh at oneself is a great skill and strength!

Aims

- To engage in physical activity and fun
- 'encourage everyone to use their voices'
- To build group cohesion

Materials

Just the group!

Method

Stand where all the children can see you.

Ask them to stand together in a group, facing you.

You will be asking the children to copy these commands, given with appropriate actions, and followed by a chorus.

1. "Thumbs up!"
2. "Thumbs up, elbows together!"
3. "Thumbs up, elbows together, knees bent!"
4. "Thumbs up, elbows together, knees bent, hips out!"
5. "Thumbs up, elbows together, knees bent, hips out, chin up!"
6. "Thumbs up, elbows together, knees bent, hips out, chin up, tongue out!"
7. Etc, until the children realise that it is all a joke.

Follow the commands with the 'Celtic' chorus, which can be pronounced however you wish, e.g. "arr-oo-chee-ka". Its main purpose is to be a rhythmic chant.

Thus:

Leader: "Repeat after me, and copy what I do."
"Thumbs up!" (raising thumbs)
Children: "Thumbs up!" (raising thumbs)

Leader: "Here's the chorus, now all join in."
"Arruchica arruchica arruchica-ca
All together: Arruchica arruchica arruchica-ca"

Leader: "Thumbs up! Elbows together!"
Children: "Thumbs up! Elbows together!"
All: "Arruchica arruchica arruchica-ca
Arruchica arruchica arruchica-ca"

Leader: Thumbs up! Elbows together! Knees bent!"
Children: "Thumbs up! Elbows together! Knees bent!
All: "Arruchica arruchica arruchica-ca
Arruchica arruchica arruchica-ca"

Leader: "Thumbs up! Elbows together! Knees bent! Hips out!"
Children: "Thumbs up! Elbows together! Knees bent! Hips out!"
All: "Arruchica arruchica arruchica-ca
Arruchica arruchica arruchica-ca"

Leader: "Thumbs up! Elbows together! Knees bent! Hips out! Chin up!"
Children: "Thumbs up! Elbows together! Knees bent! Hips out! Chin up!"
All: "Arruchica arruchica arruchica-ca
Arruchica arruchica arruchica-ca"

Leader: "Thumbs up! Elbows together! Knees bent! Hips out! Chin up! Tongue out!"
Children: "Thumbs up! Elbows together! Knees bent! Hips out! Chin up! Tongue out!"
All: "Arruchica arruchica arruchica-ca
Arruchica arruchica arruchica-ca"

Follow-on Activity 2

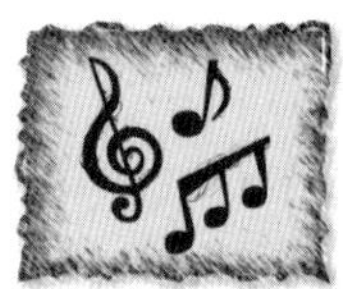

Story Soundscape

This story takes us to a variety of landscapes with many different characters. These all lend themselves to creating a 'Story Soundscape'. The aim of this activity is to create a version of the story with sound effects (although not necessarily formal music; don't be afraid of this exercise if you cannot play an instrument).
A soundscape may be done separately, or may accompany a telling of the story.

Aims

- To engage particularly with children who have a strong musicality but are verbally quiet. This exercise allows them to express ideas, thoughts and feelings and to participate fully in the story without having to talk.
- To encourage children to consider the moods and emotions in the story
- To give children the freedom to explore and enjoy playing with sounds and rhythms
- To encourage sensitivity to the spoken word, and the auditory associations and visual images which a story can evoke

Materials

Anything that the children suggest, or may be keen to improvise, including

- Percussion and other instruments (e.g. rain-stick, shaker, drum, bells, thunder-maker, thumb piano, lyre)
- Everyday objects, such as plastic bottles, newspapers, pens and rulers
- Body percussion (drumming of hands or feet, clapping, etc.)
- Mouth music, and oral sound effects (hissing, whooshing, etc.)

Method

Ask the children to consider the main elements of the story (see 'Story Skeleton' at the beginning of this chapter):

- The characters: Finn, the Fianna, Goll MacMorna, the Young Hero, the Shipwright, the Tracker, the Climber, the Gripper, the Thief, the Listener, the Marksman, the Young Hero's wife, the baby, the two little boys, the Giant, the Wolfhound, the two pups.
- The action: fast or slow, exciting or calm
- The settings: the beach, the sea, the boat, the Young Hero's home, the Giant's island tower
- The moods: dread and terror, grief and fury, relief and joy

Invite each child (or group of children) to pick an instrument and explore what sounds it can make. Then ask the children to show their instruments one at a time. (Except for the one being discussed, all instruments should be placed on the floor so they cannot be fiddled with.) Ask to hear what kind of sound each instrument makes, and what kind of emotion, mood or action it might suggest.

Discuss what sounds and instruments may be evocative for each part of the story. Each character may be assigned a particular instrument or refrain. For example, a drum roll might represent the Giant whenever he appears, or three brisk rings on a triangle might represent the Thief.

Children who play a formal instrument may also join in. Some children not experienced with a formal instrument may enjoy playing a single chord or note either at dramatic moments, or as a cue.

You and the children may decide to have sound effects or music for parts of the story only. Or you may choose to render the whole story in sound, without accompanying words.

Select which parts of the story should have sound effects or music, and map them out (coloured pens are useful to indicate different groups of instruments). Agree on how much the children should play and at what volume and tempo.

A conductor and a storyteller need to be appointed.

Ensure everybody has their instruments ready, and knows their entry points.

It works well for space to be left between the speaking and the 'sounds', rather than have the teller competing with the music.

The soundscape can be recorded and then listened to again.

If you have chosen to create a soundscape without any spoken words, it can be interesting to record this and then play it to children who didn't hear the story being told, and ask them to guess what it was about.

Follow-up Activity 3

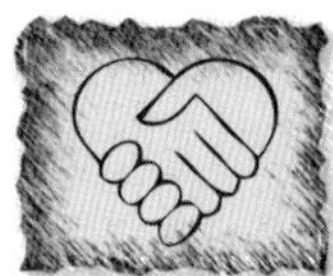

What are You Best at in the World?

In the story Finn McCool asks his new helpers "What are you best at in all the world?". He is seeking to discover which skills and qualities each Helper might be able to share with others. Ask the children, "What would *you* say to Finn if he came into the room now and asked this question?"

Aims

- To help each child to identify a skill or quality which they feel they possess, and so enhance self-esteem
- To acknowledge that different skills and qualities can be valuable and that everyone has something to offer
- To build group cohesion and 'get to know one another'

Materials

Just the group, seated in a circle

Method

Ask the children if they can recall the names and skills of Finn's Helpers, referring back to the story text if necessary.

Then pose the question, "What would you say to Finn McCool if he came into the room now and asked 'What are you best at in all the world?'" In other words, "What skill or quality makes you special?"

Some children may find this a difficult question to answer, so they can be asked if they would like some help from the rest of the group. In this case, anyone with a suggestion might put their hand up, and the child in question can choose who they would like to answer. (In this way, the child whose qualities are being discussed retains a sense of control within the group.)

Encourage children to be precise about their skill or quality. For example, if they offer 'football', ask which position they play, e.g. striker, winger, defender or goalkeeper. If a child says "Smiling a lot", this could be amplified into a personal quality of being optimistic, or having a positive outlook, etc.

Encourage aspiration. The skill may be something which a child may be working on, or would like to achieve, rather than one already mastered.

Promote the use of colourful and lyrical language, such as metaphors and similies.

Each child can be encouraged to make up a 'name' for themselves, for example, 'Rebecca the Rainbow Chaser', might be suggested by a girl who saw herself as being optimistic and good at art.

Once children have considered their responses, they can share them with the group.

This exercise can be followed by an art activity where each child makes a poster with their character name and skills, as well as a picture.

It is worthwhile keeping a note of all the responses and names. Later, these can be used in creating a 'Blessing' (see 'The Good Goodbye', Follow-up Activity 3 - Give a Blessing).

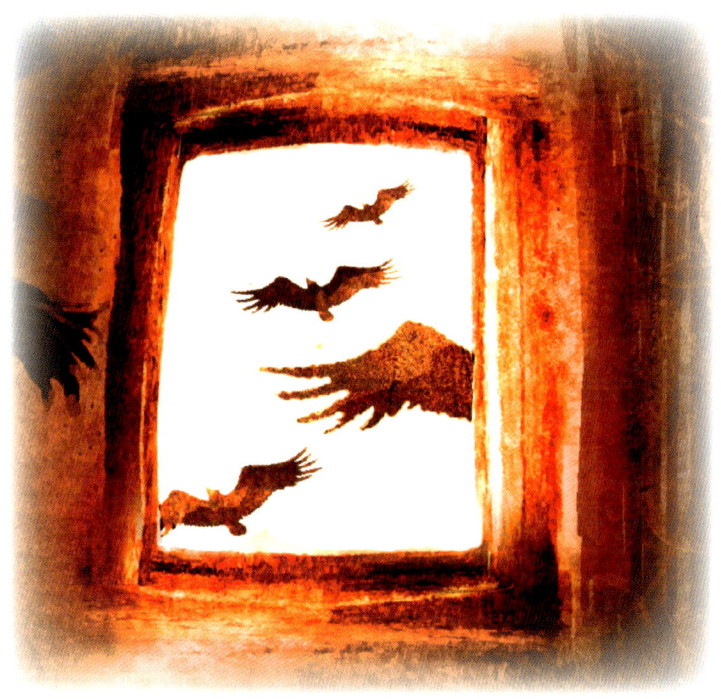

THE SEVEN RAVENS

Introduction

Stage Primary 1 (age 5) upwards

Synopsis
A longed-for baby girl is born, but is weak. Her father curses his seven sons in a moment of anger and misunderstanding. The sons become ravens and are not seen again, to their father's regret. When the girl grows up she discovers that she has seven brothers and sets out to find them. Through perseverance and sacrifice she is able to undo the curse and bring them home.

Background
This is a Brothers Grimm story with a strong female protagonist. It tends to create a calm or thoughtful mood in children.

Suggested Themes

- How a child may feel responsible for sorting out family problems
- Family sorrows and secrets
- Resolve, courage and perseverance despite setbacks
- Finding help from unexpected sources
- The power of family relationships

Skeleton

1. A longed-for daughter is born to a king and queen who already have seven sons.
2. Because the baby is frail, the King sends his eldest son for water to baptise her.
3. All seven sons race to the well, but in their haste, drop the vessels into the water. They are too scared to return to their father empty-handed.
4. The King loses his temper at the delay and curses them to become ravens.
5. The daughter grows up and learns that she has seven absent brothers.
6. The Princess confronts her parents, who say that her brothers' absence is the will of heaven.
7. Against her parents' wishes, the Princess resolves to find them. She is given a blessing by her parents, and a ring with the family crest. She also takes bread, water and a stool.
8. She journeys to the end of the world and beyond, visiting the sun, moon and stars.
9. The stars reveal that her brothers are now ravens, and live in a castle at the summit of Glass Mountain.
10. The Princess is given a piece of wood to open the castle door, and sets off on a hazardous climb.
11. On reaching the castle door, she realises that the wood-key is lost.
12. She finds a knife, and cuts off her smallest finger, which unlocks the castle door.
13. The Princess meets a little man laying a table for seven, and tells him that she is searching for her raven brothers.
14. The man says that his masters will return shortly, and the Princess meanwhile tastes food from each plate, and wine from each goblet.
15. Into the seventh goblet, she drops the family ring.
16. Seven ravens fly through the window, and the Princess hides. They sense that a human has tasted their food and wine. When the seventh raven sees the ring, he realises that the human is their sister.
17. The Princess reveals herself, and so breaks the spell.
18. They all return to their father and mother to celebrate their reunion.

THE SEVEN RAVENS

Long-ago, in a far-off land, there was a great celebration at the Palace. For the King and Queen, who already had seven fine sons, at last had a daughter. The couple had been blessed, so all their subjects were overjoyed.

But what the people did not know was that the baby was very thin and weak and the royal doctors feared she might not live. The King in his panic tried to think of ways in which this precious little bundle could be protected. The doctors prescribed potions, the Queen was given food to maximize the goodness in her breast milk, and the King decided that spiritual protection would best be achieved not only by prayer but also by immediate baptism.

He went to the room where all seven sons were anxiously pacing and waiting to hear if there was anything which they could do to help. They so wanted to do something useful! The King asked the eldest son to go quickly to the spring and draw some water to use in the baptism. All seven sons took off at great speed, grabbing jugs, cups, bowls and pitchers - anything that could carry water. They pushed and shoved and jostled, eager to please their father. In their haste, they bumped into each other, and all the vessels dropped down into the well. They were afraid to return to the Palace empty-handed, so they stood around the well, contemplating their father's wrath.

Meanwhile, back at the Palace, the King was becoming more and more angry waiting for his sons. He fumed, "Surely they have found something else to do which they deem more important than fetching this water. They are playing some game, no doubt. Can they do nothing right?"

As time passed, the King became more agitated as he thought of those strong healthy boys dallying and doing nothing to help their frail little sister. He wrung his hands and his face reddened. He almost had steam coming out of his ears!

In a moment of madness he spat out the fatal words, "I curse my sons! I curse them to be ravens!"

After a few minutes, a flapping of feathered wings was heard overhead. As the King and Queen looked out, they counted one, two, three, four, five, six, seven ravens, all as black as coal, circling above the Palace. They disappeared into the misty horizon. The King felt sorry, but did not know how to undo what he had done.

The sons were never heard of nor seen again. Years passed, and the little girl grew bigger and stronger. No one ever mentioned the missing brothers, although the King and Queen harboured a silent secret sorrow in their hearts. They took comfort in the joy brought to them by their daughter.

After many years, on her birthday, the Princess was sent to a quiet wing of the Palace while a surprise celebration was prepared. There she overheard two women of the court talking. "Aye, the princess has turned out fair!" said one woman.

"But 'tis a pity that her seven brothers have been lost for her sake," replied her companion.

A puzzled frown fell over the young Princess's face, and she vowed to challenge her parents to tell her the truth. That night she asked if she did indeed have seven brothers, and if so, where had they gone? The King and Queen told her that it was the will of heaven that they had not seen them since she was a baby. She looked into their eyes, wondering if this were true.

The Princess mourned the loss of her brothers and vowed to find them, whatever the cost to herself. Her father and mother tried to dissuade her but she was determined. At last they let her go with a blessing, "May the love in your heart give you the strength to travel with the bravery of a lioness, the surefootedness of a donkey and the shrewdness of a fox."

The Princess took with her a ring which her father and mother had given to her with the family crest on it. She also carried bread for hunger, water for thirst and a small stool for fatigue.

So she set out and journeyed on and on, but she came to the end of the world and still had not found her brothers. She climbed up into the sky and visited the sun, but the terrible heat was too much for her. She did not feel safe there.

Then she came to the moon, which was cold and lonely, and where she did not feel safe. She quickly went on and reached the stars. The stars seemed friendly as they twinkled, glittered and sparkled, saying, "Can we help you?"

The girl was pleased that at last she had found some help. She told the stars of her search, and sat on her stool to drink and eat.

The brightest star of all said, "Your brothers have been turned into ravens because of an enchantment and they live in a castle on the peak of Glass Mountain. When you reach the door, it will be locked, but take this piece of wood and with its help you may open the door." She wrapped the wood in her handkerchief and put it carefully into her pocket.

When the Princess reached Glass Mountain she climbed, she clambered, and she scrambled up its slippery slope. She felt elated when at last she stood at the castle door with its big brass lock. Eagerly she hunted for the wood in her pocket, but her heart sank when she unwrapped the handkerchief and realised that it was empty. She had lost the precious piece of wood during her climb.

The Princess then found a knife on the ground, and snatching it up, cut off her pinkie so that she could pick the lock with that. Her finger was exactly the right size. Resolutely she opened the huge door and walked down the corridor. She reached a large room with a long dining table.

A little man was setting out seven plates and seven goblets. When he noticed the Princess he asked, "Can I help you?"

She explained that she was searching for her seven brothers who had been turned into ravens.

"The Masters will return at any moment," said the man. He continued preparing the table for a meal. The girl was so hungry that she tasted the food from each of the seven plates and sipped red wine from each of the seven goblets. Into the seventh goblet she dropped the ring which her father and mother had given her. Then, with a flutter of feathers and a flash of black, seven ravens flew through the open window at the end of the room.

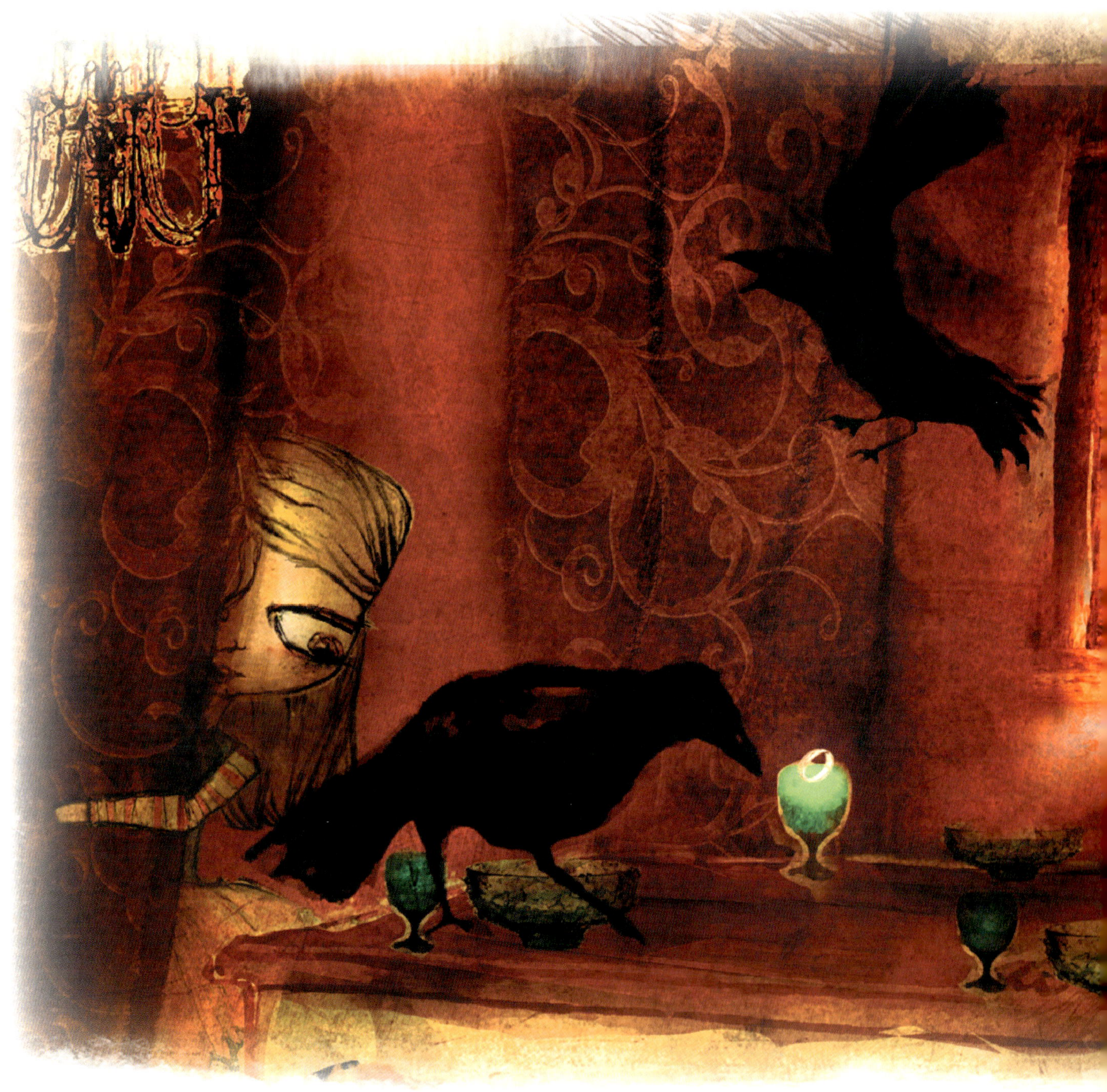

Although the Princess was amazed, she thought quickly and hid behind a screen. The ravens began to eat and drink. One by one they said, "This food has been tasted by human lips, and this wine has been touched by human lips."

As the seventh raven drained his goblet, he saw the ring, recognised it immediately, and declared, "The human is our long lost sister! If only she would come and set us free!" Hearing these words, the Princess leapt from behind the screen.

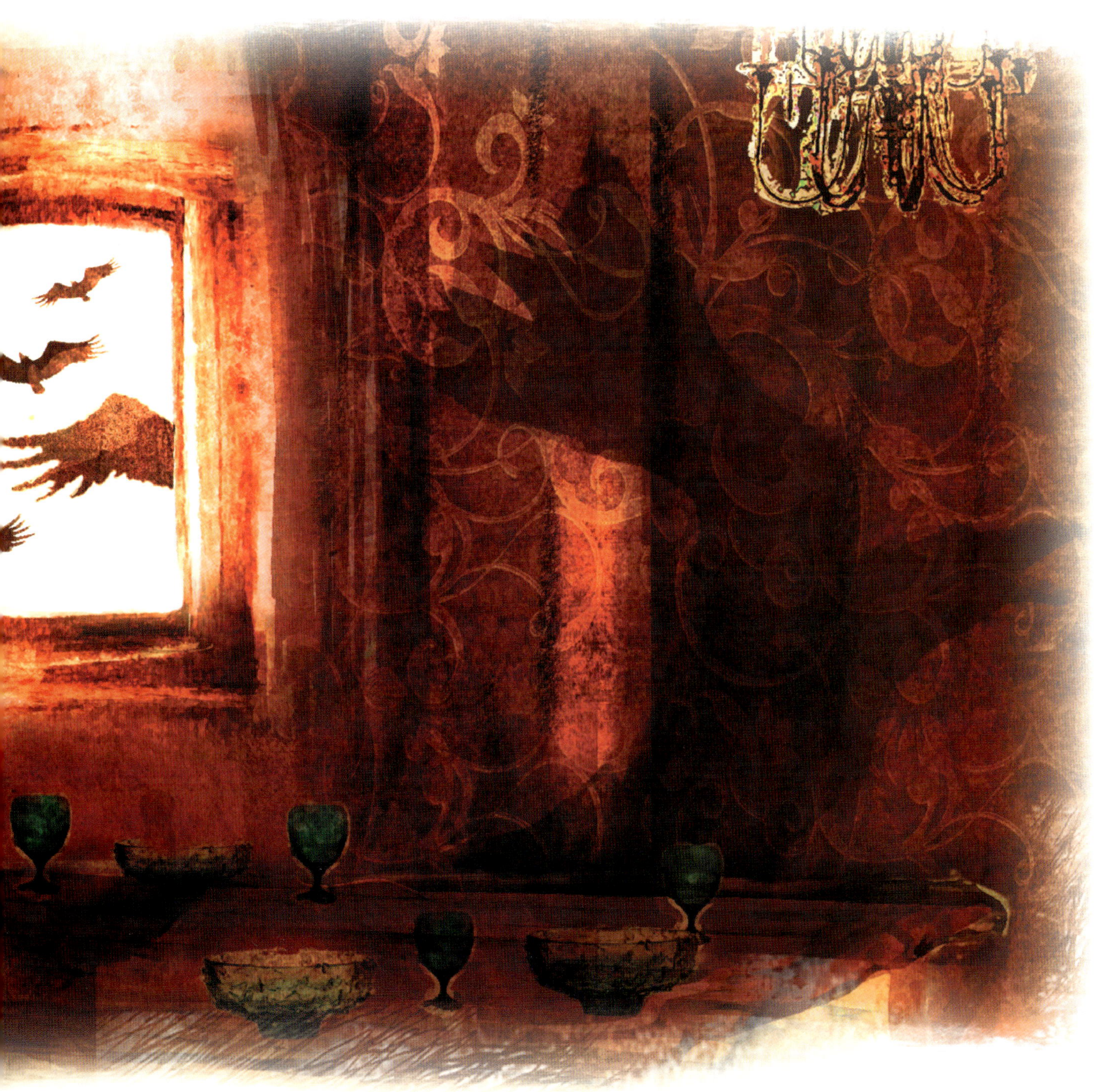

"I am your sister!" she cried. With that, the spell was broken and seven fine men stood before her. They embraced and returned together to their parents' palace to celebrate their reunion.

Follow-on Activity 1

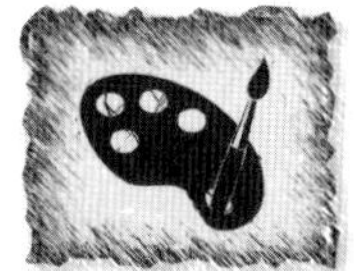

Story Sticks

This is a simple but popular method of learning a story. Various materials are tied to a stick, showing the main points of the narrative in chronological order.

Besides being a fun hands-on activity, making story sticks is a great way for children to learn a story and explore its structure. The sticks can then serve as prompts in telling the story. Each child's stick may look different, and it need only make sense to the owner.

This activity can be done by children reprising 'The Seven Ravens'; or creating their own original story (see next, Follow-on Activity 2 – Story-making with Objects); or creating a personal story (see 'Tatterhood', Follow-on Activity 2 – Personal Stories).

Aims

- To help children visualise the story and think in images and colours instead of words
- To provide an active, tactile approach to learning a story
- To understand the sequence and structure of a story

Materials

- A cane (such as bamboo or beading), or a stick from outdoors, approx. 45 cms in length, for each child
- Wool, sheep's fleece, fabric
- Pipe-cleaners, ribbon, string
- Buttons, beads, feathers
- Scissors

Method

Help the children to identify the main points of the story to be represented on their sticks. (See 'Story Skeleton' at the beginning of this chapter.)

Encourage the children to recall any other details they can think of, and to add these to their sticks. No two sticks need look alike, even if they tell the same story.

Children can be supported to think creatively and figuratively rather than literally. Different colours and textures can be used to express different story elements. For example, a piece of silky, purple fabric might represent the King, and white lace might represent the baby Princess.

Buttons and beads can be threaded onto a pipe cleaner and then twisted onto the stick. Other materials may be tied on with a simple knot (glue is not needed).

Using the story sticks, the story can then be retold in pairs, or segments of the story can be told by different children in a group. It may be useful for someone other than the teller to hold the stick, leaving the teller's hands free to make gestures.

The sticks can also be used to decorate a room, either hanging from the ceiling or across a window, or displayed in a large vase or bucket.

Follow-on Activity 2

Story-making with Objects

In this activity, children use a variety of objects as springboards to create their own stories. At first, some children may struggle with allowing their imaginations to flow, but the objects will help. Conversely, some children's imaginations may flow in all directions. Explaining the basic structure of a story, in terms of beginning, middle and end, can help children to achieve a more coherent narrative.

With the inspiration of the objects, and with an awareness of narrative sequence, children's responses can be surprising.

Aims

- To ignite the imagination with the use of tangible objects
- To work effectively with others
- To foster creativity and a sense of 'anything is possible'
- To encourage storytelling skills, especially the ordering of information
- To promote listening and talking

Materials

Collect a variety of little objects, some everyday and some more special, e.g.

- a feather
- a beautiful bead
- a teddy bear
- an interesting perfume bottle
- a foreign coin

Keep the objects in a container that will inspire some curiosity, such as a pirate chest, a shiny bag, or a woven basket.

Method

After telling the story 'The Seven Ravens', introduce the concepts of making up a story, and of story structure, explaining that each story has a beginning, middle and end.

Divide the children into groups of three, and invite each child in the group to choose an object from the collection. Ask the group to work together to create a story that includes all three objects. Suggest that the stories last for about three minutes.

Encourage each child to take part in the telling of the story (one child may take the beginning, another the middle, and a third the end). The children may first rehearse the story with each other, and then tell it to the bigger group.

Follow-on Activity 3

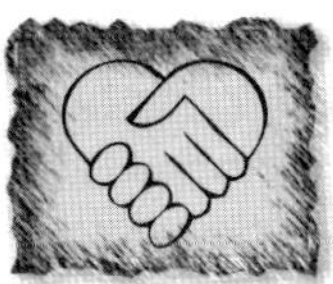

Give a Blessing

Blessings were used traditionally in many cultures and were considered very precious. There are many different types of blessing. Some may celebrate individual qualities, while others may wish general good fortune. As in 'The Seven Ravens', blessings were often given to people setting out on a journey. It was hoped that the blessing would give the traveller protection and good luck.

The natural world can inspire many different images, similes and metaphors, and is often the basis for traditional blessings.

This activity, in which blessings are composed, delivered and received, can be used effectively at times of transition or ending. Many children find such times challenging, leading to emotional or behavioural issues. Ceremony and ritual can alleviate the negative aspects of an ending, making it meaningful and positive.

Aims

- To promote a feeling of shared experience in the group
- To value each person's unique qualities
- To provide a positive experience of a transition or an ending
- To show how powerful and precious words can be
- To introduce the practice of thinking carefully about words, and of composing and drafting before writing out a final version

Materials

Scrap paper to draft blessings on:

- Card, ribbon and coloured writing pens
- Optional: flowers and candles (**note**: permission might be needed for the latter)

Method

Highlight the blessing from 'The Seven Ravens' story: "May the love in your heart give you the strength to travel with the bravery of a lioness, the surefootedness of a donkey and the shrewdness of a fox."

Explain the background to blessings, and possible occasions for their use.

For this activity, blessings may either be composed by the practitioner for individual children, or by the children for each other.

It is a good idea to do a first draft on scrap paper and then a fair copy on card.

Once written in their final form, a ceremony can be held to exchange blessings.

More detail about composing and presenting blessings follows:

Blessings composed by the practitioner
At the end of a period of contact, the practitioner can write a blessing for each child. It can be an appropriate and powerful gift: heartfelt, affirming and unique to each child. The practitioner may know the subject well and be able to highlight their qualities and strengths in the blessing. However, if this is not the case, then this exercise can be preceded by the 'What are You Best at in the World?' exercise ('Finn McCool', Follow-on Activity 3).

Here are two examples. For Bob, who says he is good at building,

> *May you build your life on a strong foundation, on rock and not sand.*
> *May you have the wisdom of the third little pig, who built her house out of bricks, not straw or sticks.*
> *May the big bad wolves flee into the forest when they are met with your fearlessness and quick wits.*

For Rebecca, who says she is good at art,

> *May your paint palette always be full of all the colours of the rainbow.*
> *May you learn to paint life in all its vibrant colours.*
> *May you discover the sunshine and the rainbows which always follow the rain.*

Blessings composed by the child
Alternatively, children may write a blessing for each other. Names can be drawn from a hat in order to decide who writes for whom. It may be helpful to provide an example from a traditional source, such as this old Celtic blessing.

> *May the road rise up to meet you,*
> *May the wind always be at your back,*
> *May the sun shine warm upon your face,*
> *May the rain fall soft upon your field,*
> *And until we meet again,*
> *May God hold you in the palm of his hand.*

For children needing more structure, a template may be given.

> *May you have the* _____ [quality] *of* _____ [a time of day],
> *May you have the* _____ [quality] *of* _____ [a place in nature],
> *May you have the* _____ [quality] *of* _____ [type of weather],
> *And may you always have the* _____ [quality] *of* ______ [an animal or bird].

Presentation of blessings
Once the blessings have been composed on scrap paper they can be carefully copied either directly onto a piece of coloured card, or else onto a decorated piece of paper, perhaps using coloured pens. It can be extra special to write the verse on a piece of paper and then insert it into a decorated folded card, fixing it with a ribbon.

A ceremony can be held to give out the blessings. The room can be decorated with flowers, and perhaps a candle lit for each person. As each name is called, the author of a blessing then reads it aloud for that person. The card is handed over, hands are shaken and then the receiver extinguishes his or her candle. This continues until each person has been given their blessing. This process can be moving, and engages children deeply if done in a reverential and special way.

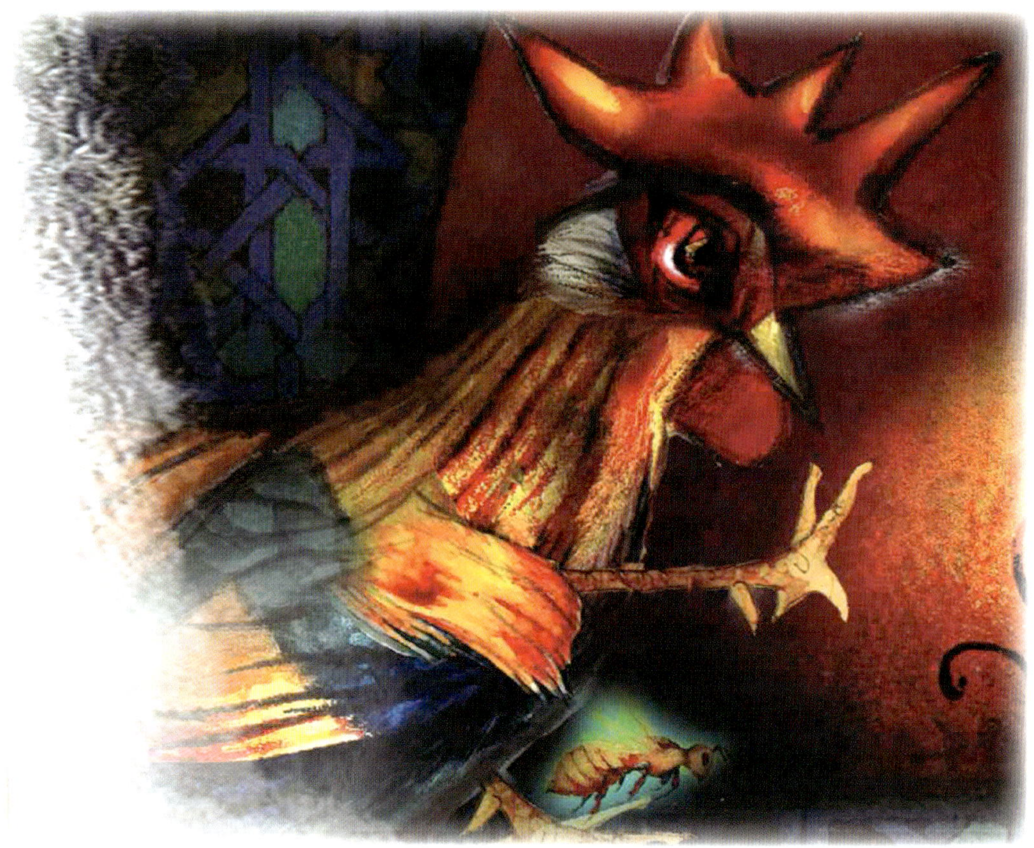

THE COCKEREL AND THE SULTAN

Introduction

Stage Primary 1 (age 5) upwards

Synopsis
A cockerel finds a golden penny and hopes to give it to his poor mistress, but a greedy Sultan takes the penny from him. The cockerel tries to get it back, and the Sultan attempts to dispose of him. The cockerel persists until the Sultan surrenders the penny.

Background
This is a version of a traditional story from Turkey.

Suggested Themes

- Life is sometimes unfair
- It can be difficult to stand up to people who are bigger or more powerful
- We can overcome adversity by using our wits
- Persistence can bring success
- Resilience is a great strength

Skeleton

1. A cockerel lives with a poor old lady and some hens.
2. He finds a golden penny and wants to give it to the old lady.
3. The Sultan takes the penny from him.
4. The cockerel follows the Sultan to the Palace, demanding his penny. The Sultan commands his guards to throw him into a well where he drinks all the water.
5. The cockerel returns to the Palace, but is thrown onto a fire, which he puts out with the water he has swallowed.
6. The Sultan has him thrown into a beehive, where he swallows all the bees.
7. The cockerel returns to the Palace, and the Sultan doesn't know where to throw him next!
8. The Sultan shoves him down his pantaloons and the cockerel spits out the bees.
9. The bees, trapped in the pantaloons, sting the Sultan.
10. The Sultan surrenders the penny to the cockerel, who gives it to the old lady.

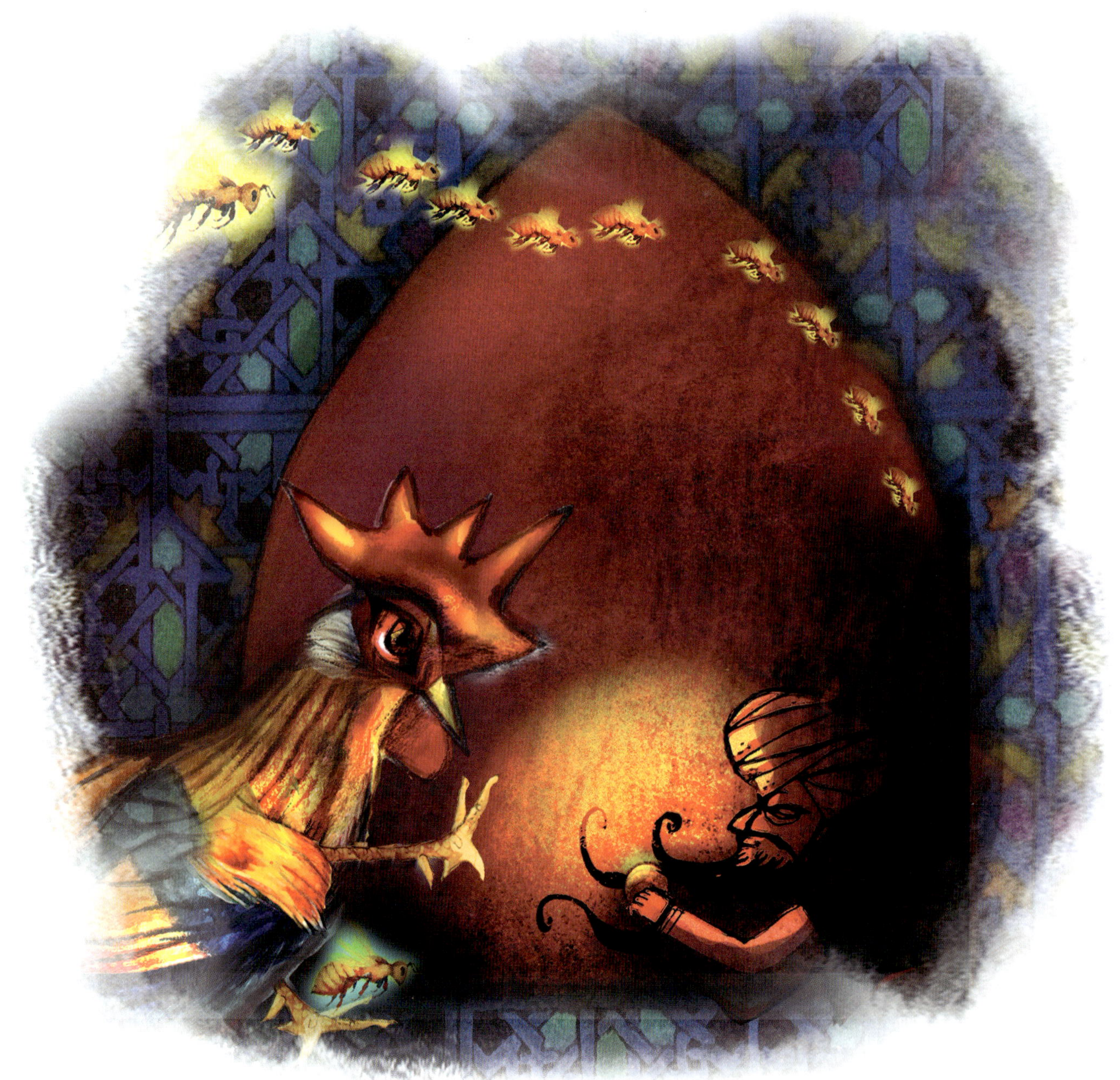

THE COCKEREL AND THE SULTAN

Once, in the far away land of Turkey there dwelled a poor old woman. She lived in an old shack and her clothes were all tattered and worn. She kept three chickens, but her pride and joy was the cockerel. Now, the cockerel was very good at looking after the hens and the old woman. As he searched among the dirt and stones, he often found useful things - a worm for the chickens to eat or a bone that the old woman could use as a needle.

One fine morning the cockerel was scraping around the yard as usual when he suddenly gave a loud and excited cry, “Cock-a-doodle-doo! Treasure, treasure! I have found a golden coin for my old lady.”

At that very moment, the Sultan of the land passed by, wearing baggy purple pantaloons and a beautiful, silk-embroidered vest. On his feet he wore curly-toed shoes and on top of his big, proud head he wore a purple turban. The Sultan was a very greedy man and when he saw the golden coin in the cockerel's beak he snatched it, saying, "I am the Sultan of this land, so that belongs to me." He marched off, out of the yard, through the town, and into the Palace.

"Well," thought the cockerel, "that will not do." So he followed the Sultan as fast as his little legs would carry him, out of the yard, through the town, and into the Palace. He flew up to the window, shrieking, "Cock-a-doodle-doo! Give me back my penny!"

The Sultan was angry. He looked the cockerel straight in the eye and growled, "Guards! Throw him down the Royal Well."

The Guards did as they were bid and threw the cockerel into the deep well. Splash! He landed in the water at the bottom and he did not like it one bit! The cockerel's wings were so wet that he couldn't fly. But then he had an idea. He opened his beak and sucked up all the water until the well was dry, and so were his feathers. Then he flew up to the Palace window and again shrieked at the Sultan, "Cock-a-doodle-doo! Give me back my penny!"

The Sultan was furious. He looked the cockerel straight in the eye and growled, "Guards! Throw him onto the fire!"

So they did. The cockerel did not like the hot fire one bit! But then he had an idea. He opened his beak and spat all the water from the well onto the flames and put them out. Then he flew up from the ashes to the Sultan's window and again shrieked, "Cock-a-doodle-doo! Give me back my penny!"

By now the Sultan had steam coming out of his ears! He looked the cockerel straight in the eye and growled, "Guards! Throw him into the Royal Beehive!" So they did. Now, you know who lives in the Royal Beehive - bees! The cockerel looked at the bees and he had an idea. He thought that they might make a good snack. So he opened his beak and pecked up the bees. They were delicious – ten, fifty, one hundred, one thousand bees! Then he flew up to the Palace window and screamed at the top of his cockerel's voice, "Cock-a-doodle-doo! Give me back my penny!"

The Sultan was so livid that he did not know where to put the cockerel next! In desperation he grabbed the cockerel by the neck and shoved him into his silk pantaloons. The cockerel didn't like being inside the Sultan's trousers one bit so he began spitting out all the bees from his tummy! But the bees were now trapped in the trousers and became angry. Of course, when bees are angry what do they do? Yes, the bees stung the Sultan well! He began to hop and skip from one foot to the other in agony. The Guards struggled not to laugh as they watched the Sultan do a very strange little dance. At last he released the bird and said, "Cockerel, you win! I will give you back your penny!"

The cockerel took the coin in his beak and marched off, out of the Palace, through the town and home into the yard. He proudly handed over his golden penny to the old lady with a "Cock-a-doodle-doo!"

His mistress was overjoyed and said, "Thank you, Cockerel. Now we may live in comfort for the rest of our days."

Follow-on Activity 1

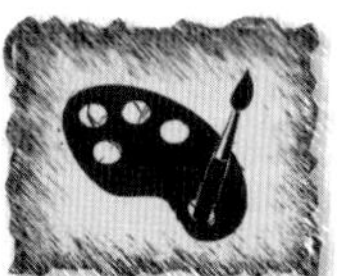

Envelope Puppets

This enjoyable activity is suitable for all ages. The puppets can be very simple, or more elaborate.

Aims

- To create props which help children participate in telling the story
- To stimulate the imagination
- To have fun making an object

Materials

These may vary depending on the characters chosen.

- New or used envelopes (A4 or A5), opened on the narrowest side
- Coloured paper, tissue paper, crepe paper
- Fabric, wool, braid, ribbons, etc.
- Googly eyes, buttons, or bottle tops
- Felt pens
- Glue and scissors

Method

Ask the children to consider the characters in the story: the old woman, the hens, the cockerel, the Sultan, the Guards, and the bees.

Encourage the children to consider the main features of the characters they have chosen to make, e.g. a cockerel looks like a cockerel because of its beak, wattle, comb, small eyes, and feathers. It may be useful to search the Internet for images.

To make a puppet: first, fold back the top corners of the envelope to make a 'head' shape. Add any specific features, and decorate according to individual taste.

Ask the children to help retell the story using their puppets, inserting their hands into the decorated envelopes and animating them when their character enters the story. They can also be encouraged to join in with some of the lines, either all together or one at a time. The refrain "Cock-a-doodle- doo! Give me back my penny!" can be chorused by the whole group.

Follow-on Activity 2

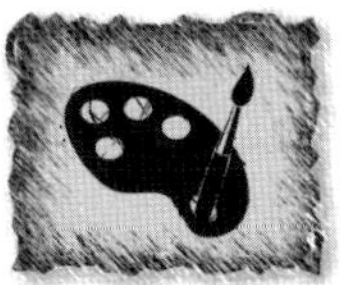

Story Sticks

This is a simple but popular method of learning a story. Various materials are tied to a stick, showing the main points of the narrative in chronological order.

Besides being a fun hands-on activity, making story sticks is a great way for children to learn a story and explore its structure. The sticks can then serve as prompts in telling the story. Each child's stick may look different, and it need only make sense to the owner.

This activity can also be used by children creating their own original story (see 'The Seven Ravens', Follow-on Activity 2 – Story-making with Objects), or creating a personal story (see 'Tatterhood', Follow-on Activity 2 - Personal Stories).

Aims

- To help children visualise the story and think in images and colours instead of words
- To provide an active, tactile approach to learning a story
- To understand the sequence and structure of a story

Materials

- A cane (such as bamboo or beading), or a stick from outdoors, approx. 45 cms in length, for each child
- Wool, sheep's fleece, fabric
- Pipe-cleaners, ribbon, string
- Buttons, beads, feathers
- Scissors

Method

Help the children to identify the main points of the story to be represented on their sticks. (See 'Story Skeleton' at the beginning of this chapter.)

Encourage the children to recall any other details they can think of, and to add these to their sticks. No two sticks need look alike, even if they tell the same story.

Children can be supported to think creatively and figuratively rather than literally. Different colours and textures can be used to express different story elements. For example, a piece of silky, purple fabric might represent the Sultan, and a gold button might represent the golden penny.

Buttons and beads can be threaded onto a pipe cleaner and then twisted onto the stick. Other materials may be tied on with a simple knot (glue is not needed).

Using the story sticks, the story can then be retold in pairs, or segments of the story can be told by different children in a group. It may be useful for someone other than the teller to hold the stick, leaving the teller's hands free to make gestures.

The sticks can also be used to decorate a room, either hanging from the ceiling or across a window, or displayed in a large vase or bucket.

Follow-on Activity 3

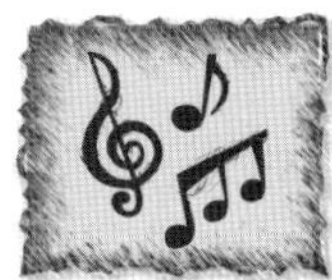

Story Soundscape

This story takes us to a variety of landscapes with many different characters. These all lend themselves to creating a 'Story Soundscape'. The aim of this activity is to create a version of the story with sound effects (although not necessarily formal music; don't be afraid of this exercise if you cannot play an instrument). A soundscape may be done separately, or may accompany a telling of the story.

Aims

- To engage particularly with children who have a strong musicality but are verbally quiet. This exercise allows them to express ideas, thoughts and feelings and to participate fully in the story without having to talk.
- To encourage children to consider the moods and emotions in the story
- To give children the freedom to explore and enjoy playing with sounds and rhythms
- To encourage sensitivity to the spoken word, and the auditory associations and visual images which a story can evoke

Materials

Anything that the children suggest, or may be keen to improvise, including:

- Percussion and other instruments (e.g. rain-stick, shaker, drum, bells, thunder-maker, thumb piano, lyre)
- Everyday objects, such as plastic bottles, newspapers, pens and rulers
- Body percussion (drumming of hands or feet, clapping, etc.)
- Mouth music, and oral sound effects (pecking, crowing, buzzing, etc.)

Children who play a formal instrument may also join in. Some children not experienced with a formal instrument may enjoy playing a single chord or note either at dramatic moments, or as a cue.

Method

Ask the children to consider the main elements of the story (see 'Story Skeleton'):

- The characters: the hens, the old lady, the cockerel, the Sultan, the Guards, the bees
- The action: fast or slow, exciting or calm
- The settings: the yard, the Palace, the well, the fire, the beehive
- The moods: furious, threatening, defiant, challenging, triumphant

Invite each child (or group of children) to pick an instrument and explore what sounds it can make. Then ask the children to show their instruments one at a time. (Except for the one being discussed, all instruments should be placed on the floor so they cannot be fiddled with.) Ask to hear what kind of sound each instrument makes, and what kind of emotion, mood or action it might suggest.

Discuss what sounds and instruments may be evocative for each part of the story. Each character may be assigned a particular instrument or refrain. For example, a clashing of cymbals might represent the Sultan whenever he appears.

You and the children may decide to have sound effects or music for parts of the story only. Or you may choose to render the whole story in sound, without accompanying words.

Select which parts of the story should have sound effects or music, and map them out (coloured pens are useful to indicate different groups of instruments). Agree on how much the children should play and at what volume and tempo.

Songs can be added, particularly as a refrain. For example, a song could be created for the cockerel to sing when asking for his penny.

A conductor and a storyteller need to be appointed.

Ensure everybody has their instruments ready, and knows their entry points.

It works well for space to be left between the speaking and the 'sounds', rather than have the teller competing with the music.

The soundscape can be recorded and then listened to again.

If you have chosen to create a soundscape without any spoken words, it can be interesting to record this and then play it to children who didn't hear the story being told, and ask them to guess what it was about.

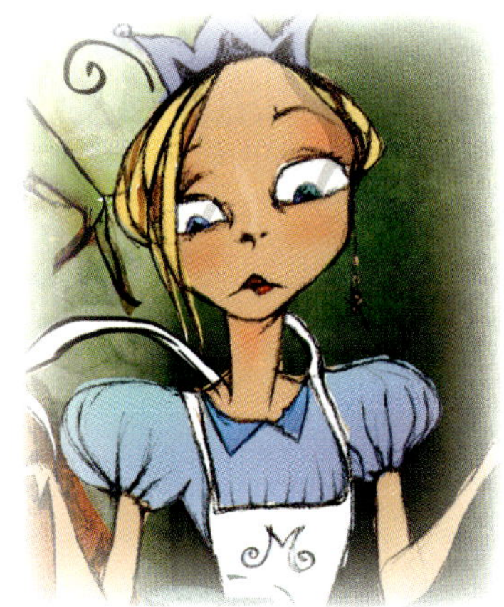

JACK AND MARIGOLD

Introduction

Stage Primary 3 (age 7) upwards

Synopsis
A young woodcutter, Jack, sets off to find his fortune. When a king urges Jack to marry his spoilt daughter, Marigold, Jack refuses. But he suggests that Marigold accompany him as he ventures into the woods. Marigold is a difficult companion, spurning the fruit offered by apple and pear trees. Leaving Jack, she is captured by Witch Wash-a-Dish, who chains her up and makes her wash mountains of dishes. Jack rescues her and they flee, but the apple and pear trees refuse to hide Marigold. The fir tree gives her protection and the Spirit of the Woodland grants it evergreen leaves. The apple and pear trees must lose their leaves in autumn as a punishment. Jack and Marigold marry and live happily ever after.

Background
This story has an exciting plot, which includes a climactic battle with a cruel witch. There is humour and irony, as well as some serious themes. The characterisation is very strong: likeable, principled Jack; exasperating but redeemable Marigold; and the truly horrible Witch Wash-a-Dish. The story also resonates with a creation myth, for which the seeds are planted early on, but which only becomes explicit towards the end. It is a popular story, perhaps for all these reasons.

Suggested Themes
- Respecting the natural world, rather than taking it for granted
- Being thankful for what we have, rather than complaining
- Material possessions are less important than good values
- Being prepared to listen to wise advice, even if it means changing our minds
- The importance of being kind and respectful to others
- Why some trees lose their leaves in autumn, and why some are evergreen

Skeleton

1. Jack, a young woodcutter who lives with his poor mother, sets off to seek his fortune.
2. He visits a neighbouring kingdom, where the king is desperate to find a husband for his spoilt daughter, Marigold. The King offers Jack her hand, but neither Jack nor Marigold is keen.
3. Jack says that Marigold can join him for a week, while he ventures into the woods and lives off the land, to see if they are compatible.
4. Marigold goes with Jack, but she is reluctant to leave her comfortable life. They explore the woods for food, finding an apple tree and pear tree.
5. Marigold offends the trees by refusing their fruit.
6. At nightfall, Jack suggests that they shelter in a woodman's hut, but Marigold storms off, determined to return home.
7. Jack tries to warn her about Witch Wash-a-Dish, who lives in the woods, but Marigold pays no heed.
8. Marigold is followed through the woods and captured by the witch. She is chained to the kitchen sink, and forced to wash mountains of dishes under the watchful eye of the witch's cat.
9. Marigold accidentally breaks some dishes and is beaten by the witch.
10. Marigold regrets her earlier selfish, spoilt behaviour, and longs to see Jack again.
11. Jack rescues Marigold and tells her to hide in the trees.
12. The apple tree and then the pear tree, remembering Marigold's earlier rudeness, refuse to hide her from the witch. A fir tree, however, does give Marigold shelter.
13. The witch pursues Marigold, and the apple tree and the pear tree point out Marigold's path to her. But the fir tree does not betray Marigold.
14. The witch runs on through the woods in search of Marigold, and is never seen again.
15. Jack and Marigold, safe at last, hug each other. Marigold apologises for her earlier behaviour.
16. The Spirit of the Woodland appears, and declares that the apple tree and the pear tree should have helped Marigold. So from now on they must lose their leaves every winter. But the fir tree will remain evergreen.
17. Jack and Marigold return to the King's palace, where they fall in love, have fourteen children, and live happily ever after.

JACK AND MARIGOLD

There was once a laddie called Jack. He lived with his mother, who was a poor widow. He worked in the woods all around as a woodcutter. But he cared for the trees and only cut down those that were sick or broken. He then chopped the wood, loaded it into a handcart and sold it to people who needed to burn wood in their fires. In those days everyone burned wood in their fires. One day Jack thought that he would like a change of scene, and so he decided to set off to seek his fortune in the big wide world. When he asked his mother what she thought of his plan, she said, "Good for you, Jack!" and made him a bread-piece for his journey.

Well, unbeknown to Jack, in the next kingdom there was a king who had only one daughter. Her name was Marigold. She was the most spoiled little brat you could ever meet and the King was fed up with her. He wanted her to marry and have some grandbairnies for him, but she found fault with every suitor who was brought before her. The King said, "You are far too fussy, critical and selfish when it comes to other folk. Well, madam, I have had enough! The very next person who walks through that door, you will marry!"

With that there came a knock at the door. The King grinned, rubbed his hands together, and shouted, "Come in!"

In walked Jack. He bowed, saying, "Good morning, Your Majesty! Do you have any wee jobs that need doing?"

"Oh yes!" said the King. "I've a muckle big job. You can marry that wee maiden over there and take her off my hands!"

"Hold on a minute," said Jack. "I was thinking of chopping wood or doing a bit of painting. Call me old-fashioned, but I always thought that when I got married I would at least know the lassie, and hopefully love her! I've never seen this lass before in my life."

"Well, that's all good and well. Aye, very romantic! But last time I looked I was the one wearing the crown. That makes me the king and the one that everybody wants to please. So do as you're told and marry her!"

"Ahem," interrupted Marigold, clearing her throat. "Is anyone going to ask me what I think?"

"No, we are not," snorted the King. "We have heard enough from you to last us a lifetime!"

"Well," said Jack, "I'll tell you what I'll do. I'm off on an adventure into the woods. I'm going back to nature, to live off the land. So I'm willing to take her with me for a week. But after that, if we don't get along, then I'll bring her back. Do we have a deal?"

"I suppose you can't say fairer than that. Off you go, and see if you can sort her out a bit," sighed the King.

Marigold pulled a face. "If I am to go then I need to pack my white trainers, my Wii, my Nintendo, my iPod, my hair-straighteners, my . . . "

"No, no, Marigold, you don't need any of that stuff. We'll be going back to your roots, come as you are. Let's go." So off she trudged with her face trippin' her.

Before long Marigold started girning. "I'm hungry," she moaned. "Is there a McDonald's around here? I fancy a cheeseburger and a milkshake."

"No," smiled Jack. "There is nothing like that around here. But I can show you the feast that can be found in the woods if you just know where to look. See, here's an apple tree!" Jack approached the tree, and recognising him as a friend, she lowered her branches so he could reach her rosy red apples. "Help yourself," said Jack to Marigold.

Marigold looked at the apples and screwed up her face. "Yuck! They are probably sour and full of maggots!" The apple tree was offended by this and lifted up her branches.

"Never mind," said Jack, "we'll find you something else to eat." Soon they came to a pear tree whose branches were heavy with golden orbs. Jack stepped close to the tree and she too knew him, so she lowered her branches. "Here, Marigold, delicious pears," said Jack.

But Marigold scowled and said, "Yuck! Fusty old pears? No thanks!" The pear tree was offended, and lifted her branches. On they went through the woods, until it began to get dark and Marigold complained that she was tired.

"There's a woodcutter's hut further on, where I'll make a bed for you out of grass and straw," said Jack.

"A bed of straw? I am a princess and am used to a bed of goose feathers!" screeched Marigold.

"I am trying my best, Marigold, but you are pretty hard to please!" shouted Jack, who was usually a very patient lad.

"Well, I've had enough of this so-called adventure! I'm going home to my feather bed, and my daddy," she shrieked.

"You can't leave now," said Jack, flatly. "Everyone knows these woods are meant to be haunted at night."

"That's a load of gossip, and I don't care about gossip," scoffed Marigold, turning on her heel.

"But they say that Witch Wash-a-Dish haunts these woods." called Jack, urgently. But Marigold was heading off down the path, retracing her steps.

"Marigold, come back!" pleaded Jack. But there was no telling her. She was off!

As Marigold walked she felt a little nervous, so she stuck out her chest to make herself feel braver. Moonlight cast strange shadows through the branches of the trees onto the path ahead. The woods seemed alive with all kinds of noises. [*Note to the practitioner: ask the children to make some noises.*] Marigold thought she could hear footsteps behind her. She stopped, and looked over her shoulder. But there was nothing there. She took a deep breath. Probably just a rabbit! So Marigold walked on. But soon she thought she heard footsteps again. She stopped, and looked over her shoulder. There was nothing there. Probably just a fox!

So on she walked. Suddenly, she felt one hand gripped around her waist and another slapped across her mouth. She was lifted up and tossed like a feather in the wind, to the north, the south, the east and the west. Then she was flung down onto a cold, stone floor in what seemed to be a kitchen.

All Marigold could see when she looked up was a sink full of dirty dishes. Then she saw an old woman, and she shrieked, “Are you Witch Wash-a-Dish?”

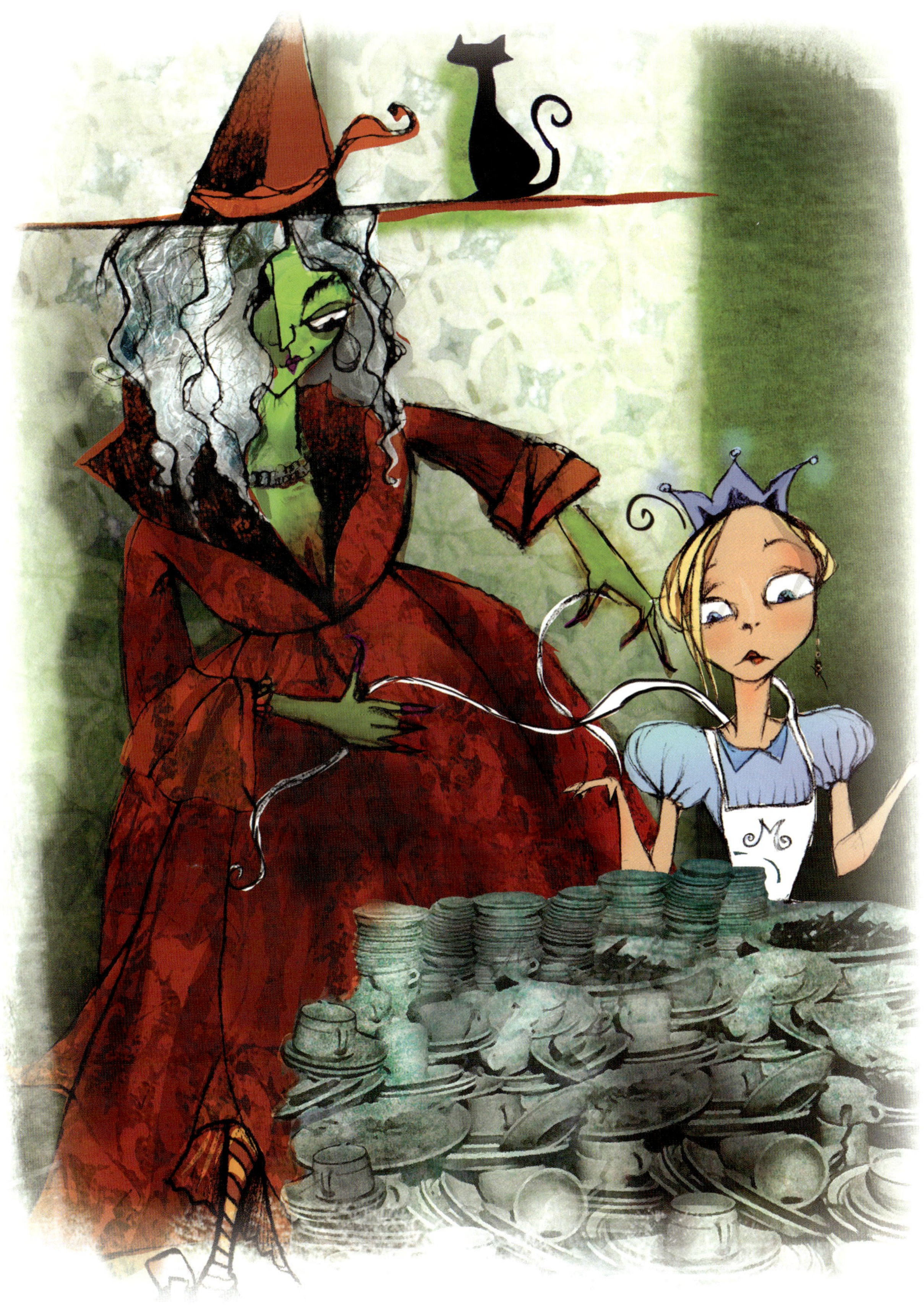

"Why, yes, my dear," replied the witch. 'Does my reputation precede me? Do you know why they call me Witch Wash-a-Dish?'

"Is it because you like washing dishes?" Marigold ventured.

"No!" cackled Witch Wash-a-Dish, "It's because I *never* wash dishes. I get children like you to do it for me."

"Well," Marigold explained politely, "this time you've made a mistake because I never wash dishes either. You see, I'm a princess. I wouldn't know how!"

"Oh, you'll soon learn, my dear. And if you so much as crack or chip my precious china dishes then I'll have your guts for garters and I'll grind your bones. Then I'll scatter them in my garden to make my plants grow bonny!" said the witch, grimly.

With that the witch tied a chain around Marigold's ankle and clamped her to the sink. Then she left her old black cat in the corner to keep an eye on things (for whatever a witch's cat sees, the witch can also see in her mind). And then she was gone.

Marigold started sniffling as she filled the sink with hot soapy water. "Oh dear, I wish I'd listened to Jack. I can't do dishes, they are so slimy and slippery . . . Oh!" With a loud crash, a plate slid from her grasp and smashed on the stone floor. The witch flew back, as quick as a flash. She beat her soundly, and Marigold cried all night.

The next day she began washing again, wishing that she had not been so clumsy the day before, nor so selfish the day before that, when . . . CRASH! Another plate fell to the floor.

"If you break one more dish," screamed the witch, "then I'll have your guts for garters." The witch beat her soundly once more, and Marigold cried all night

Early next morning Marigold began washing the dishes again. She was longing to see Jack. Just then, who should pop up at the window but Jack! "Oh Jack! I'm so glad to see you!" squealed Marigold. "You've got to get me out of here, right now! The witch says she's going to kill me if I break one more dish!"

"Let me think," said Jack, rubbing his chin with his eyes rolling skywards. "I know! I'll go fishing."

"Fishing! How can you think of going fishing at a time like this!" yelled Marigold. [*Note to the practitioner: ask the children, "Why might Jack want to go fishing?"*]

Jack disappeared and returned ten minutes later with a little silvery trout which he held up at the window. When the cat sprang to eat the fish, Jack caught it in a big sack. He tied the top of the sack, trapping the cat.

The witch knew immediately that something was wrong. She started running back through the woods on her stiff old legs. Jack leapt through the window and began filing the chain around Marigold's leg. While the witch ran, Jack filed; and while Jack filed, the witch ran. Just as the witch reached the cottage door, Jack broke through the chain and he and Marigold jumped out of the window.

"Quick, Marigold! Find a place to hide in the trees!" shouted Jack, sliding into the branches of a tree. Marigold ran for her life, and was relieved when she saw the apple tree. She panted,

Apple tree, apple tree, please hide me,
For witches and fairies do find me,
And Auld Wash-a-Dish will brack ma bones,
And grind them atween twa marble stanes.

But the apple tree said, "Aren't you the one who said that my fruit was sour and full o' maggots! No, I winna hide ye!"

"Oh!" exclaimed Marigold. She ran on and soon came to the pear tree. She pleaded,

Pear tree, oh pear tree, please hide me,
For witches and fairies do find me,
And Auld Wash-a-Dish will brack ma bones
And grind them atween twa marble stanes.

But the pear tree said, "Aren't you the one who said that my fruit was old and fusty! No, I winna hide ye!"

"Oh!" exclaimed Marigold. She ran on and came to a fir tree. She begged,

Fir tree, oh fir tree, please hide me,
For witches and fairies do find me,
And Auld Wash-a-Dish will brack ma bones,
And grind them atween twa marble stanes.

The fir tree opened up her branches and hid Marigold from sight. Hot on Marigold's heels came Witch Wash-a-Dish. She ran up to the apple tree and said, "Have you seen a spoilt wee brat come running through these woods today?"
"Aye," said the apple tree, pointing with her branches. "She went that way."

"Hee hee!" said Witch-Wash-a-Dish, and on she hirpled.

Then she saw the pear tree and said, "Have you seen a selfish little madam come through these woods today?"

"Aye," said the pear tree, pointing with her branches. "She went that way."

"Hee hee!" squealed the witch, and on she scurried.

Then she saw the fir tree and she asked, "Have you seen a hoity-toity lassie come running through these woods today?"

"No," said the fir tree, "I've seen no one."

So Witch Wash-a-Dish ran on through the woods, on and on, and has never been seen since. When all seemed safe, Jack crawled out of his hiding place and called for Marigold. She emerged, and said, "Oh Jack, I wish I'd listened. You were right, I am stubborn and hard to please. But no more, I promise." Then the two gave each other a hug.

A tinkling music filled the air and in a bright shaft of light the Spirit of the Woodland was revealed. "Apple tree," she said sternly, "when this maiden asked you for help today, did you give it?"

"No, no - I don't suppose I did," mumbled the apple tree, bowing her branches.

"And you, pear tree, did you give this lass help when she most needed it?" asked the Spirit.

"Well, no - not really," admitted the pear tree, shamed.

"From this day forth at this time of year, you apple tree, and you, pear tree, will lose all your leaves and so will spend the coldest darkest days of the year with bare branches. You, fir tree will remain green all the year round," the Spirit proclaimed. And so it is to this day.

And what of Jack and Marigold? They went back to the King's palace, where they did get to know each other. Indeed, they fell in love, married, and gave the King fourteen grandchildren to bounce upon his knee. And of course they lived happily ever after!

Follow-on Activity 1

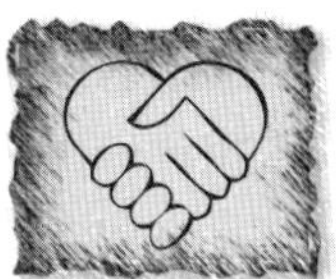

My Hero

In the story, Jack is the obvious hero. He sets out to find his fortune, but, being principled, declines to marry the King's daughter, Marigold because he doesn't know her, yet alone love her. He has a good sense of humour, and isn't overawed by the King. He is wise in the ways of nature, and of the woods. He is kind to the prickly Marigold, and mostly patient. He is resourceful and daring, as when he rescues Marigold from the terrifying witch. He is forgiving, and is glad to be friends with Marigold despite all the mistakes she has made.

It's worth mentioning that Marigold, while not a 'conventional' hero in the same way as Jack, also has some positive and heroic qualities: she stands up to her father when he tries to marry her off; she can be determined; and she can be brave. Perhaps most importantly, she eventually admits to her mistakes, and decides to be wiser in future. And that takes a special kind of courage and strength.

We all have heroic qualities inside us. We don't need to have special powers and wear a cloak to be a hero! Nor do we need to perform daring deeds.

This activity, which can be either oral or written, or a mixture of both, asks the children to consider three questions in turn: 'What deeds did Jack perform which made him a hero?'; 'What qualities does Jack have'?; and 'What qualities and actions in your own life might be seen as everyday heroism?'

Aims

- To encourage reflection about ourselves and our positive attributes
- To realise that being a 'hero' is as much about how we lead our lives every day, and about our everyday deeds, as it is about meeting extraordinary challenges
- To emphasise that we can ultimately shape our own destiny: both by being true to ourselves in difficult circumstances, and, when opportunity arises, being ready to move forward or to change

Materials

- Pencil and paper
- Flip chart or whiteboard

Method

The children will be asked to consider three questions in turn:

- What deeds did Jack perform which made him a hero?
- What qualities does Jack have?
- What qualities and actions in your own life might be seen as everyday heroism?

These questions are designed to build towards a realisation that it is Jack's personal qualities rather than just his deeds which make him heroic.

'What deeds did Jack perform which made him a hero?'
Ask the children to discuss this question in pairs, aiming for at least three deeds. Then bring the group back together. Jack's deeds might include:

> He refused the king's demand that he marry his daughter.
>
> He found Marigold after she had been kidnapped by Witch-Wash-a-Dish.
>
> He took time to think of a sure way to trap the witch's cat, instead of panicking.
>
> He filed the chain from Marigold's leg, even though the witch was approaching and he could have run away himself.

Write the children's ideas on a flip chart or whiteboard.

'What qualities does Jack have, and how were these shown?'
Again, ask the children to discuss this question in pairs, aiming for at least three examples. There may be a wide variety of responses, such as:

> He is honest: he tells the king he cannot marry someone he doesn't know or love.
>
> He thinks ahead: he plans where to stay in the woods.
>
> He respects nature: he values the fruits that the trees offer to him.
>
> He is thoughtful: he looks after Marigold, seeking food and shelter for her.
>
> He is brave: he goes to the witch's cottage.
>
> He is resourceful: he thinks of an ingenious way to trick the witch's cat.
>
> He is persistent and loyal: he doesn't abandon Marigold to the witch.
>
> He is forgiving: he forgives Marigold for behaving like a 'spoilt brat'.

Write the children's ideas on a flip chart or whiteboard.

'What qualities and actions in your own life might be seen as everyday heroism?'
The focus in this third stage of the activity shifts from the story to the children's own lives. A useful bridge is to emphasise that Jack would have possessed all his heroic qualities in daily life, in little deeds, as well as in big adventures. In fact, it is because he would have been like this from day to day that he is able to handle such big challenges.

Ask the children, either in pairs or individually, to consider (and perhaps write down) three of their own 'everyday hero' qualities, with examples of how they have shown these through their actions. There may be a wide variety of responses, such as:

> I am strong: yesterday I carried out the recycling box for my Mum.
>
> I am patient: this morning I waited for my sister while she got ready for school, without getting angry.
>
> I don't give up: even though I found my maths test hard, I kept trying my best right till the end.
>
> I am kind: yesterday I made my Mum a cup of tea.
>
> I am brave: last month I went to the dentist and had an injection.

Some children might be more comfortable with a qualifier, such as:

> Sometimes I have been brave: I once rescued our cat from a tree.
>
> Sometimes I think ahead: I saved for a present for my Mum's birthday.
>
> I can be determined: when I lost my favourite hat, I looked everywhere until I found it.

Ask for volunteers to share some of their examples with the wider group.

Follow-on Activity 2

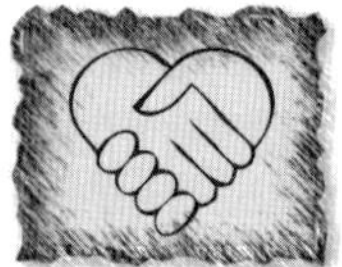

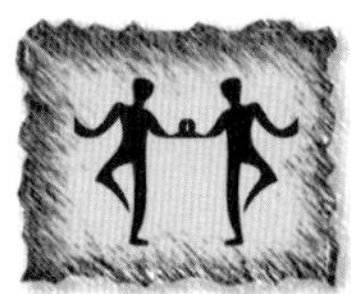

Anyone Who

In the story, Jack and Marigold come from very different worlds and have very different interests. Marigold is a spoilt princess, and Jack is a sensible woodsman. Jack finds Marigold difficult to get along with, while Marigold shows no appreciation of Jack's knowledge and skills. But as they get to know each other better, and fight the witch together, they become best friends, and even end up married!

When we make friends, it is good to find out what the other person likes. It shows that you are taking an interest in the other person and you can find out what you have in common. This game helps us to do just that.

Children love this game, which shares some similarities with 'musical chairs'. The main challenge is getting them to stop!

Aims

- To help the children to find common ground and build group cohesion
- To encourage quiet members of the group to talk
- To encourage the whole group to mix
- To enhance skills in listening and talking
- To encourage cooperation
- To provide physical movement

Materials

- The group
- A chair for each participant in the group, less one

Method

Make a circle of chairs, on which the children are seated, but with one chair missing.

One participant stands in the centre and asks, 'Anyone who . . . ?', finishing the line with a characteristic which is likely to apply to some of the group.

An example might be, 'Anyone who . . . has brown eyes?'. Then all those with brown eyes must stand up, and find a new seat. The asker of the question must also find a seat. This must be done in a cooperative fashion.

The person who is left without a seat then asks the next 'Anyone who . . . ?' question.

Other questions might include things that people like or are wearing, such as: 'Anyone who likes pizza?', or 'Anyone who is wearing a white shirt?'

Children can be encouraged to decide on their question before it is their turn to ask.

Encourage the children to think about the cooperation that is needed in this game both to make it work and to avoid anyone being hurt in the hunt for chairs.

Follow-on Activity 3

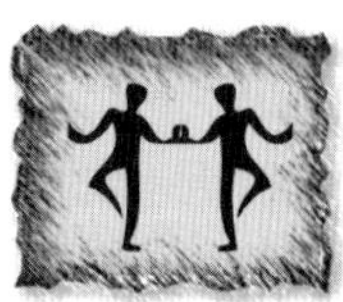

Harvesting a Story

In 'Jack and Marigold' the characters journey through the woods. Woodcutter Jack is at home in this environment, but Princess Marigold finds it strange and threatening. Jack respects the natural world, but Marigold is dismissive and insulting. So rude is she to the pear tree and the apple tree that they refuse to hide her from Witch Wash-a-Dish. But the fir tree takes pity on her, and Marigold comes to value both Jack and the natural world which is so important to him.

This outdoors activity encourages the children to use natural garden or woodland materials as inspiration for story-making. In small groups, they are asked to make up a story, depicting it on the ground with the materials they have 'harvested'. They are then asked to tell their story to the larger group, which moves from site to site, listening to each illustrated story in turn.

This activity echoes '"The Seven Ravens", Activity 2, Story-making with Objects', but is also inspired by the environmentally-conscious 'land art' movement, which uses natural materials to create temporary installations.

It is useful to visit the outdoor area first and ensure that there is enough appropriate material for the children to 'harvest' for their illustrated stories.

Allow one to one-and-a-half hours for this exercise, and plan it for a fine day!

Note: Some ground rules may need to be set, such as staying within a well-defined area, not picking flowers from flowerbeds, not damaging trees, etc.

Aims

- To create a story with a natural illustration
- To explore the world around us and connect with nature
- To be creative and use imagination
- To work as part of a team
- To develop storytelling skills

Materials

- Use of a garden or wooded area, with some clear ground space, and adequate natural materials in the vicinity
- Natural materials, such as leaves, cones, twigs, grasses, wildflowers, and stones
- A bag or basket in which materials can be collected

Method
Explain to the children that the aim of this activity is three-fold: to make up their own stories in small groups, drawing inspiration from surrounding materials; to illustrate these stories by creating their own 'land art' on the ground; and then to tell their stories, in turn, to the rest of the group.

Remind the children, briefly, of the story 'Jack and Marigold', and of how a story has a beginning, middle and end. It also has a character (or characters), and a setting (or settings).

Divide the children into groups of three.

Invite them to explore the area and 'harvest' available natural materials for their story-making.

Once a selection of material has been found, ask the children to work in their own group space, coming up with their story idea. Each child may make their own character which can then be woven together into a group story.

If no story idea emerges, encourage the children to just make a picture with the materials. The materials might prompt a picture of a character, or a setting, that leads to a narrative.

The story should be about three minutes long. The ground image accompanying it may be any size.

Follow on with a storytelling event, with each group telling their story to a mobile audience, in situ.

The images can be photographed and then left to be carried away by the wind.

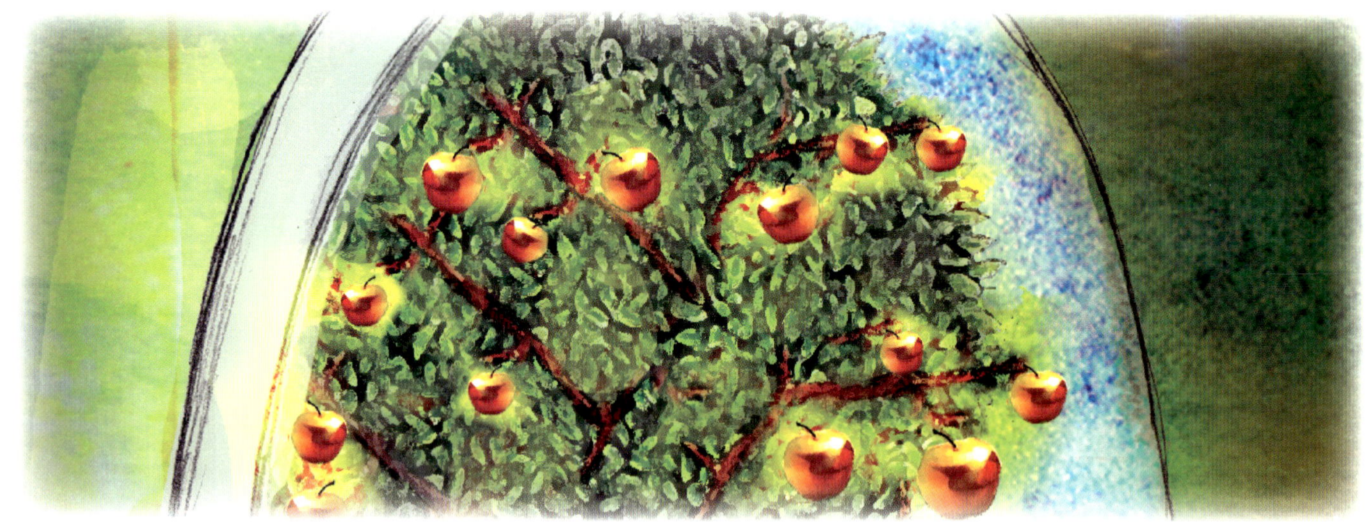

ONE-EYE, TWO-EYES, THREE-EYES

Introduction

Stage Primary 2 (age 6) upwards

Synopsis
Two-Eyes is a stepdaughter in a family with strange eyes. She is lonely and ill-fed until she adopts a pet goat which she later learns can provide her with a feast on request. Enraged, her stepmother has the goat killed. Grieving, Two-Eyes buries its heart. From the heart's grave springs a tree with golden apples. A passing prince sees the apple tree, falls in love, and takes Two-Eyes away to a new life.

Background
Originally collected by the Brothers Grimm, this is a Scottish version of the story. The emblematic apple tree, with its golden fruit, echoes Greek, Norse and Celtic myth. Today, variations of this story can be found as far away as India.

Suggested Themes

- Being an outsider, or being different
- Loneliness, and being true to oneself, even if this means being alone for a while
- The complexity of sibling relationships
- Fortitude and resilience in the face of adversity
- Coping with loss and grief
- The importance of holding onto hope for a better future, even in the darkest hour
- The benefits of listening to wise advice
- Moving onto the next chapter of life, and growing up

Skeleton

1. A young girl lives and suffers in a strange-eyed family. Her harsh stepmother has four eyes, and her step-sisters each have one eye, and three eyes. They are called One-Eye and Three-Eyes. The young girl has two eyes, and so is called Two-Eyes.
2. Two-Eyes does all the housework, and also tends the sheep and goats. She is given little food, and has to forage for nuts and berries on the hillside. She is hungry and lonely.
3. Her only friend is a little pet goat, abandoned by its mother.
4. One day, in despair, while tending the flocks on the hillside, Two-Eyes is told by a tiny man that her pet goat will provide a feast on request, if she rubs its ear and chants some special words.
5. Now, instead of starving, Two-Eyes enjoys a secret feast on the hillside each day.
6. The suspicious stepmother sends One-Eye to spy on her stepsister, but Two-Eyes sings her to sleep with a lullaby.
7. The stepmother sends Three-Eyes, who feigns sleep while peeping through one of her eyes, and so learns Two-Eyes' secret.
8. The stepmother has the goat killed.
9. Two-Eyes is distraught. Her friend, the wee man, advises her in her grief.
10. Following his instructions, she has a cry, says a prayer, and buries the goat's heart in the garden.
11. The next day, an apple tree with golden fruit has grown where the heart was buried.
12. A prince, passing by, asks to buy a golden apple.
13. The tree resists the stepmother and her daughters when they try to take fruit from its branches.
14. An apple rolls to the feet of Two-Eyes, and she is revealed as the true owner of the tree.
15. The Prince asks her to marry him, and they leave for a new life together.
16. The apple tree withers and dies, while the Prince and Two-Eyes live happily ever after.

ONE-EYE, TWO-EYES, THREE-EYES

Well, you may think your family is a little odd; most of us do! But this story is about a very strange family indeed. There were three sisters and a mother. Now, the middle sister had one eye, right in the middle of her forehead, so she was called One-Eye. The oldest sister had three eyes, one in the middle of her forehead and two on either side of her head, so she was called Three-Eyes. The mother had four eyes, one on either side of her head, one at the front and one at the back. The youngest child was a stepchild who had two eyes in the usual places and so was called Two-Eyes. The others were all jealous of her, perhaps because she looked like most people do.

Two-Eyes had to do all the hardest work in the house: cleaning, washing, and chopping firewood. At night, when the others sat down to a hot dinner, Two-Eyes was given only a bowl of cold, watery porridge.

Each morning, Two-Eyes would herd the sheep and goats up the hill so they could graze. In summer and autumn she found nuts and berries to eat, as she was always hungry. But in winter there was nothing, and all she had was cold porridge at home.

One day, a goat gave birth to a runt kid. Two-Eyes knew the little kid would be left by its mother to die. She persuaded her stepmother to let her keep it as a pet. Oh, Two-Eyes loved this kid. She carried it everywhere, she spoke to it and fussed over it; it was her best and only friend in the world.

One winter's day Two-Eyes climbed up the hill with her pet. She felt so miserable that she just sat down and cried. She sobbed until a tiny voice asked, "What's wrong wi' you, lass?"

Two-Eyes looked up and through bleary eyes saw a strange little man. She answered, "I'm hungry, ravenous. I never get much food at home."

"Well, if that's the problem," said the manikin, "then that is easily fixed. Rub your wee goat behind its ear and say, 'Bleat, little goat, bleat, and give me something good to eat.'"

Two-Eyes obeyed, and immediately, a feast of food appeared before her on a crisp, white tablecloth. Her eyes widened. There was chicken, beef, fish, salad, cakes, bread - you name it, it was there! She tore into the food and invited the manikin to do the same. Soon she was satisfied. But there was lots of food left over.

"What shall I do with all this food?" asked Two-Eyes.

"That's no bother," said the little man. "Just rub your wee goat behind the ear again and say, 'Bay, little goat, bay, and take the good food away.'"

So she did, and the tablecloth with its food disappeared as quickly as it had come.

Two-Eye's life now changed, as she was able to have a great, secret feast every day! Each night when she was offered watery porridge at home, she said, “No thanks,” and slipped off to bed.

However, the stepmother grew suspicious. She saw that Two-Eyes was looking healthy, with roses in her cheeks, a twinkle in her eye and shiny hair. She also noticed that Two-Eyes was not only refusing her porridge but also going to bed early. So one night when Two-Eyes had gone to bed she said to her daughters, “Listen here, Two-Eyes is up to something, and you must find out what it is. One-Eye, go up the hill with her tomorrow and keep your eye on her the whole time!”

Next morning, One-Eye went up the hill with Two-Eyes. At first Two-Eyes was glad of the company, until she realised that she couldn’t have a feast with One-Eye watching her. So she led One-Eye to a nice soft patch of grass and encouraged her to lie down and relax. Then Two-Eyes sang her a sweet lullaby and watched as she slowly closed her eye, and fell asleep.

Vair me oh ro van oh,
Vair me oh ro van ee,
Vair me oh ro ho ho,
Sad am I without thee.

Two-Eyes hugged her goat and rubbed it behind the ear, whispering, “Bleat, little goat, bleat, and bring me something good to eat.”

As usual, a feast appeared and Two-Eyes tucked in. Then, when she was satisfied, she said “Bay, little goat, bay, and take the good food away.” With that the food vanished.

One-Eye woke up. She stretched and yawned, saying, “Oh, have I missed anything?”

“Not at all,” replied Two-Eyes.

When they returned home the stepmother waited until Two-Eyes had refused her porridge and gone to bed early. Then she leaned close to One-Eye and asked, “Well, what did you see on the hill today?”

“Nothing, Mother,” said One-Eye.

“Nothing? Did you keep your eye on her all the time?”

“Aye, Mother. Well . . . except when I had a little nap.”

“Och, you’re useless! Right, Three-Eyes, tomorrow you will go up the hill with Two-Eyes and keep all your eyes on her the whole time!”

So the next morning Three-Eyes went up the hill with Two-Eyes. At first Two-Eyes was glad of the company, until she realised that she wouldn’t be able to have a feast with Three-Eyes watching her. Two-Eyes decided to try the same trick she had used with One-Eye. She led Three-Eyes to a nice soft patch of grass and encouraged her to lie down and relax. Then Two-Eyes sang her a sweet lullaby and watched as she slowly closed her eyes.

Vair me oh ro van oh,
Vair me oh ro van ee,
Vair me oh ro ho ho,
Sad am I without thee.

But she didn't notice that the eye on Three-Eye's forehead was still slightly open, peeking at Two-Eyes.

She grabbed her goat and rubbed it behind the ear, saying, "Bleat, little goat, bleat, and bring me something good to eat."

Again a feast appeared and Two-Eyes tucked in. Three-Eyes couldn't believe her eye! She struggled to stay calm and not jump to her feet. Instead, she pretended to be asleep and watched quietly. When Two-Eyes was satisfied, she said, "Bay, little goat, bay, and take the good food away." With that the food disappeared.

Three-Eyes pretended to wake up. She stretched and yawned, saying, "Oh, have I missed anything?"

"Not at all," replied Two-Eyes.

When they returned home the stepmother waited till Two-Eyes had refused her porridge and left the room. Then she leaned close to Three-Eyes and said softly, "Well what did you see today?"

"Oh, Mother, you wouldn't believe it! That pet goat, it gives her food. It's magic!" answered Three-Eyes.

"Is that right now? Well, we'll soon put a stop to that!" hissed the stepmother. She went outside and told the gardener to kill the little goat.

The next morning Two-Eyes got up and couldn't find her pet. She asked her stepmother where it might be, and she replied, "There will be no more wee goat, because it is dead!"

Two-Eyes was beside herself. Sobbing, she ran away up the hill. She had lost her best, her only friend in the whole world.

As she sat crying in the heather, she heard a familiar voice. "What are you greetin' for now, lass?"

Two-Eyes looked up, to see the manikin. "My wee goat is no more! My stepmother has had it killed!" she wept.

"Och, well now. That is terrible, but I'll tell you what to do to soothe your grief. You must go to your stepmother and ask for the heart of the wee goat. Take it, and bury it in the garden. Say a prayer and shed some tears. It will bring comfort, to know that your wee pal is at rest. Then you must hold your memories of the dear little goat in your heart forever."

The poor girl did as she was told. She retrieved the goat's heart; she buried it in the garden, said some prayers and shed some tears, and cherished the memory of her little friend. Then she went to bed. The next morning she woke to find her bedroom filled with an amazing golden light. Two-Eyes jumped up, thinking she had slept until the middle of the day. She looked out of her window to find the source of the light, and saw a huge apple tree growing out of the very spot where she had buried her goat's heart. The apples weren't green or red, but gold, solid gold!
Two-Eyes ran downstairs and there was her stepmother staring at the tree with her mouth wide open.

"What are you glaurin' at?" snapped the stepmother, turning on Two-Eyes. "Off you go round to the kitchen and get on with your work!"

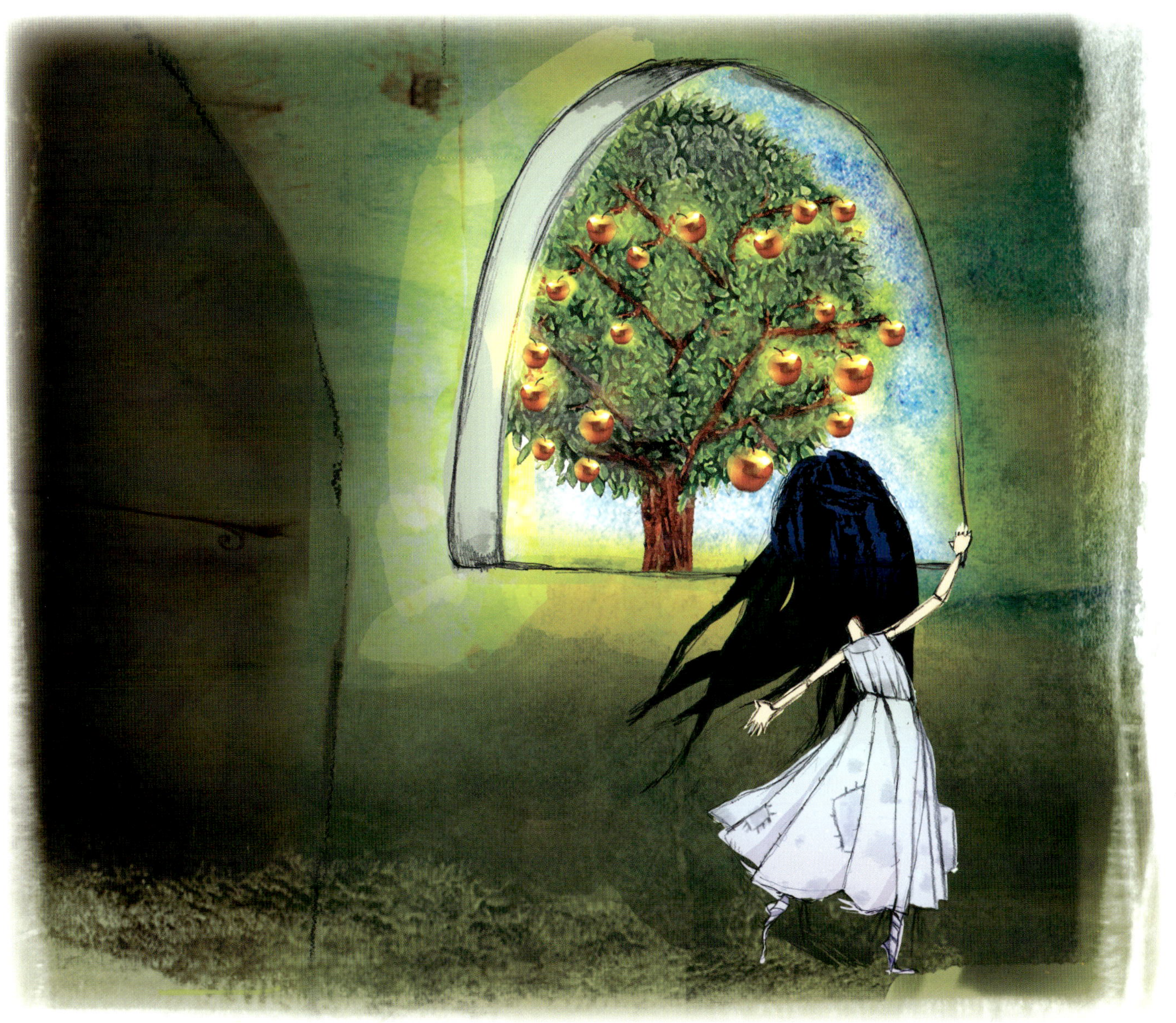

Just then a prince came riding by. He stopped when he saw the remarkable tree, his face full of wonder. "Is this your tree?" he enquired of the stepmother.

"Well, of course it is!" she roared. "It's in my garden so who else's tree would it be?"

Then she softened as the Prince asked, "May I buy one of these apples?"

"Certainly," she smiled, immediately becoming more friendly. She reached up for an apple, but all the branches of the tree shot up the trunk beyond her reach.

"It's not really your tree, is it?" said the Prince.

"Well no, it's my daughter's," the stepmother replied, coyly. She bellowed, "Three-Eyes! Come here!"

"May I buy one of these apples?" asked the Prince, politely.

"Certainly," smiled Three-Eyes.

She reached up for an apple, but all the branches of the tree flew around to the other side of the trunk beyond her reach.

"It's not really your tree, is it?" said the Prince.

"Well no, it's my sister's." So she summoned One-Eye.

"Is this your tree?" asked the prince.

"Oh yes, it is." replied One-Eye, brazenly.

"May I buy one of these apples?"

"No bother!" she beamed.

She reached up for an apple, but all the branches of the tree moved up the trunk beyond her reach. One-Eye was not going to give up easily, so she leapt on to the trunk of the tree and started to climb, grabbing at the apples. But the branches of the tree crashed down and battered her on the head! She was knocked right off the tree.

"It's not really your tree, is it?" said the Prince, looking at her on the ground.

"No," said One-Eye, rubbing her head.

Just then an apple fell from a branch and rolled down the path towards the back of the house. It stopped when it reached the feet of Two-Eyes.

"Is that your tree?" asked the Prince.

"Yes," she answered.

"May I buy one of these apples?" he asked.

"Certainly," she smiled.

She reached up into the branches and an apple fell, 'plop', into the palm of her hand. She handed it to the Prince and he looked deep into her eyes.

"Would you like to come away with me and be my bride?" he asked hopefully.

"Yes," she replied, "If you can offer me something other than watery porridge for my dinner each night . . . "

He lifted her onto his horse and the two rode away together. And the apple tree? People say that the very next day the apple tree withered and died. But Two-Eyes lived with her prince, happily ever after.

Follow-on Activity 1

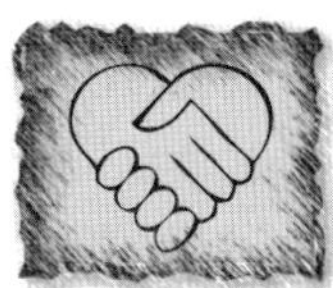

Letter-writing for Emotional Literacy

Unusually, this exercise occurs in the middle of the story-telling. The children are invited to consider the emotions of the protagonist and to imagine themselves in her situation. They express their feelings in a letter to the protagonist, and offer her some advice about how to act.

The Latin root of the word 'emotion' is 'emovere', meaning 'move out'.
This exercise shows how we can be moved to act as a result of feelings.

Aims

- To identify and empathise with the character in the story
- To learn about different emotions: what they mean and what they feel like
- To encourage the children to consider feelings before actions
- To help the children to realise that more than one emotion can be felt at the same time, for example 'sad' and 'angry'.

Materials

- Paper and pencil

Method

Before telling the story for the first time, facilitate a 'brainstorm' of different emotions and what they mean.

Then tell the story up to a point which you think illustrates emotions that you'd like the children to explore. For example, the part of the story where the stepmother has killed the little goat might help the children to consider sadness and anger. Pause the telling of the story and begin the exercise.

(continued...)

Ask the children to each write a personal letter to Two-Eyes, in the following format:

> Dear Two-Eyes,
>
> I am so sorry to hear that your little goat has been killed. If I were you I would be feeling
>
> 1. ________
> 2. ________
> 3. ________
>
> I suggest that you ____________________________ [advice for action].
>
> Yours sincerely,
>
> ____________ [signature]

Ask volunteers to read their letters to the group, so that children hear each other's ideas about feelings and action. More discussion can follow this exchange.

Continue with the remainder of the story. By now the children will be very keen to learn how Two-Eyes comes to terms with her grief, and how the narrative unfolds.

Allow time for reflection and discussion about how the story develops, compared with the children's projections.

Follow-on Activity 2

Re-telling the Story

This may seem a very simple activity. Yet it is one which children really enjoy and involves a great deal of skill.

Aims

- To boost confidence in storytelling skills, and especially in verbal expression
- To learn about story structure
- To build cohesion in a group
- To improve memory
- To develop listening skills

Materials

Just the group, seated in a circle.

Method

Encourage the children to offer ideas about the skills which might help in telling a story well. (Hint: In the chapter 'Using this Pack', refer to the section 'Telling the Story'.)

Ask the children to volunteer to tell part of the story. Invite children to put their hand up, or otherwise indicate that they would like to tell the next part. This can continue around the group until the story is finished.

There may be points where some help is needed so that the story approximates the original version. The practitioner may be sensitive in accepting different interpretations of what happened, saying, "It's interesting that you heard that in the story," rather than "That's not right". A useful question is, "Did anyone hear that part differently?"

Ensure that the children render the story in a story-telling fashion, rather than just giving an account of what happened.

If a child gives a general account, it is worth asking if any details can be recalled, such as, "What was Two-Eyes given for supper each night?", or "What sort of tree grew from the goat's heart?" Children can then be praised for their good listening skills.

Follow-on Activity 3

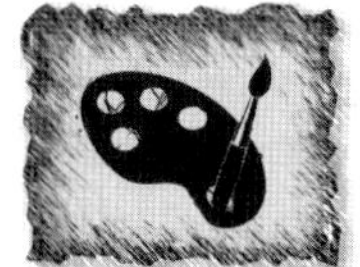

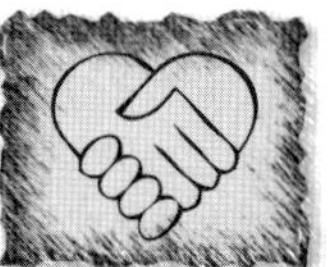

A Special Place

This activity focuses on the apple tree which springs from the buried heart of Two-Eyes' beloved goat.

The apple tree, with its fruit, is an archetypal symbol which features in many mythologies. Its significance may vary somewhat between different stories and cultures, and from person to person. It can represent the Tree of Knowledge, the Tree of Life, or the Tree of Love – or, indeed, all of these. In the tale of Two-Eyes, the tree bears apples which are golden. In Greek mythology, golden apples stand for love, and in Norse mythology they symbolise rebirth and immortality. So Two-Eyes' apple tree has a rich background!

More generally, trees are rich in life: as sources of food and as havens. Creatures live in and around all parts of a tree: amid the bark, the wood, the leaves and the roots. They have their own habitats and havens.

In this exercise, children are invited to imagine themselves living as tree-dwelling creatures. Then, on a drawn or painted image of a tree, they can create their own 'special place' (such as a nest or burrow) with craft and natural materials.

Aims

- To promote the idea that each individual (whether creature or person) is entitled to a place where they feel safe and special
- To consider how this can be achieved
- To encourage the notion of different individuals or colonies living side by side, perhaps separately, perhaps symbiotically
- To explore different textures and materials, and encourage design skills

Materials

- Sheets of paper, either large (for a group), or smaller (for individuals)
- Crayons or paints
- Cotton wool, wool, felt or fabric
- Leaves, twigs, feathers, or other natural materials
- Glue

Method

This activity can be done either in a group, using a large-scale image of a tree; or individually, on a smaller scale.

Prepare an outline of a tree on appropriate-sized paper.

Encourage discussion about trees as habitats: what kind of homes they provide, and for whom. Different creatures have different needs, and so may choose to live in a tree's roots, in its bark, trunk or branches, or among its leaves.

Ask the children to imagine themselves as tree-dwelling creatures, and, using the materials available, to make a 'special place' for themselves in the tree.

When completed, invite further discussion about the 'chosen places' which the children have made. They can

- describe them, and the materials chosen to make them
- consider the advantages and disadvantages of their choice
- decide whether they would live alone; or, if not, then who they would choose to live with them
- consider what might be added to their tree, or changed, in order to make it feel special. (Here, it might be helpful to recall that the tree of Two-Eyes was distinguished by its folding branches and golden apples.)

The pictures can then be displayed.

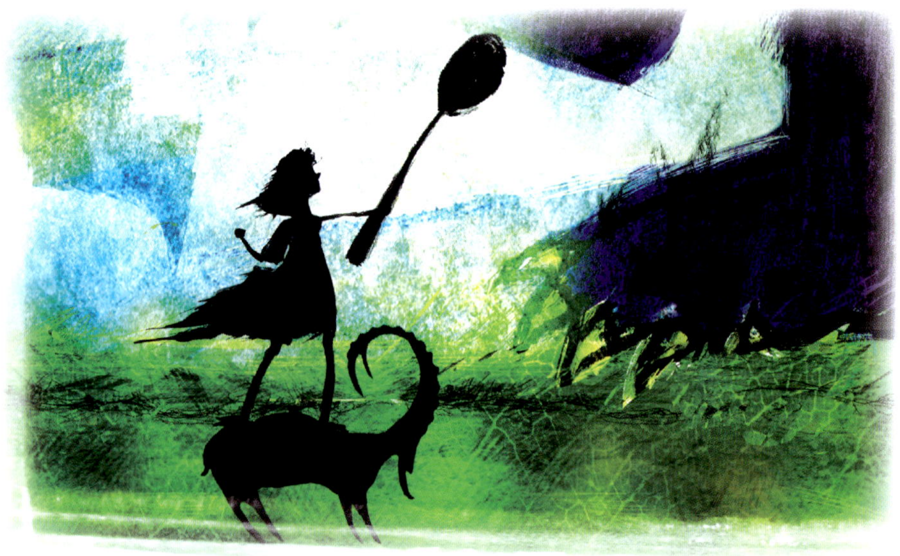

TATTERHOOD

Introduction

Stage Primary 1 (age 5) upwards

Synopsis
A bitter Queen longs to have a baby, but instead adopts a daughter, whom she neglects. Through her she finds a way to become pregnant and has twin girls. The Queen favours Lily, whom she sees as pretty, but Tatterhood grows up to be strong, smart, and brave. When gentle Lily's head is stolen by the Trolls, who leave a cow's head in its place, Tatterhood and Lily set out to recover it. Tatterhood defeats the Trolls, and then ensures that both Lily and herself marry and live happily ever after.

Background
This story, from a Norwegian source, is well known in Orkney due to the Norse connection there.

Everyone loves this story, whether they are five or eighty-five years old, and it seems to appeal equally to boys and girls. Besides being full of action, its themes are many and varied, and can be explored at different levels, depending on the listeners' responses and on the practitioner's judgement. 'Tatterhood' can work well as a 'first' story for a group.

The story raises the issue of 'a favourite' in the family, yet the sisters themselves are loyal to each other despite their different attributes, and despite the difference in how they are seen by their mother. The story also challenges stereotypes and encourages us to think about how we perceive others. It addresses the issue of 'looks', and handled carefully, can be a challenging and rewarding story. Tatterhood herself, scorning the importance of appearances, and the opinions of others, is an especially positive female role model.

Suggested themes

- Favouritism from a parent (either real or assumed)
- Sibling relationships
- The power of love and loyalty
- Standing up for what one believes in, and being true to one's self despite the opinions of others
- Being tenacious and resilient, whether enduring hardship or following a goal
- Being brave and adventurous in a hostile world
- How appearances may be deceptive, and are less important than what lies beneath
- The possibility of changing one's perceptions of others

Skeleton

1. A queen, unhappy because she has no children, adopts a girl, but fails to love her. The Queen doesn't even name the child, but just calls her 'Adopted Daughter'.
2. A servant takes pity on the lonely girl and gives her a golden ball to play with in the palace garden.
3. An urchin girl climbs over the wall to play with Adopted Daughter.
4. The Queen is furious, until the urchin explains that her mother, who works in the palace kitchen, knows of a way to be sure of having a baby.
5. The urchin's mother tells the Queen to wash herself at bedtime, and then throw the water under the bed, where two flowers will grow. One flower will be beautiful, and the other ugly. She should eat the beautiful one, but leave the other.
6. The urchin and her new friend, Adopted Daughter, leave the Queen, the palace, and the story.
7. The Queen follows the strange instructions, but can't resist eating both flowers.
8. She has twin girls: one whom she thinks looks ugly, and the other beautiful.
9. The first girl, who was born carrying a wooden spoon and riding a goat, is given a tattered cloak with a hood, so that the Queen does not have to look at her. She is named Tatterhood. The other girl is called Lily.
10. Despite their mother's attitude, Tatterhood and Lily are very close to each other.
11. Trolls approach the palace, trying to steal Christmas.

12. Ignoring the Queen's scorn, and armed with her wooden spoon, Tatterhood rides out on her goat to fight the Trolls.
13. Tatterhood defeats the Trolls. But Lily, anxious about her sister, opens the castle door. A Troll steals her pretty head and leaves a cow's head in its place.
14. Tatterhood and Lily set sail for the land of the Trolls. Tatterhood retrieves Lily's head from the Trolls' castle. Mounted on her goat and armed with her spoon, she defeats them again in battle.
15. Back at sea, and with Lily's head restored, Tatterhood calls in at an attractive-looking island.
16. She demands to speak to the King, who falls in love with Lily and asks for her hand in marriage.
17. Tatterhood agrees to the match, provided a husband is found for her as well.
18. The King persuades his son to marry Tatterhood, even though the Prince has not yet met her. A joint wedding is planned.
19. Crowds flock to the wedding procession. Lily and the King make a handsome couple, beautifully dressed and mounted on splendid horses. But Tatterhood seems to have made no effort at all. She is still carrying her wooden spoon, riding her goat, and wearing her tattered cloak. The crowd is bemused, and the Prince, now that he has met Tatterhood, is puzzled by her oddness.
20. Tatterhood asks the Prince if he has any questions for her before they are married. When he asks about her spoon, goat and cloak, she suggests that they are really a wand, a horse, and a wedding gown.
21. The Prince gradually changes his view of Tatterhood as they approach the altar, and he falls in love.
22. The double marriage takes place amid much joy.

TATTERHOOD

In the land of Norway, there was once a queen who was very miserable, and the reason for her discontent was that she had never had a child of her own. One day a servant suggested that she could adopt a child and so she did. The Queen adopted a little girl, but she did not love her. She did not even give her a name, but simply called her 'Adopted Daughter'.

The Queen was very strict with Adopted Daughter, forbidding her from playing outside the palace grounds. And so the child was very lonely, with no one to play with. One day a servant took pity on her, and gave her a golden ball. She ran out to the garden, and threw it up and caught it, again and again, until it dropped and rolled into the bushes. When she parted the bushes to search for the precious ball, she saw a dirty face, framed in matted hair, looking back at her. It was a girl of about her own age, dressed in rags. "Who are you?" she asked.

"I am an urchin child," replied the ragged little girl. "I live on the street but I heard you playing alone, so I thought I would climb over the wall and join you!"

Then the little urchin picked up the golden ball and tossed it to Adopted Daughter. They threw the ball back and forth, giggling with delight. Their laughter rippled through the air and reached the ears of the Queen.

The Queen stormed to the palace window and saw the street child. Furious, she ran down the stairs and into the garden. She shrieked at the urchin, "Get out of my garden, you piece of vermin!"

But the little girl was not afraid. She put her hands on her hips, and, cocking her head to one side, said, "You wouldn't talk to me like that if you knew what I know."

"Now what could you possibly know that would be of interest to me?" asked the Queen.

"I know how to have a baby," announced the urchin.

"Well, I think we all know how to have a baby, you silly girl!" replied the Queen.

"But this way is one hundred per cent guaranteed," said the little girl.

So the Queen invited the urchin into the palace. Once seated, the girl said hesitantly, "Actually, it's really my old mother who can tell you all about it. She works in your kitchen."

So the Queen sent for the old woman, who merely said, "Now, don't you be listening to my daughter. She's talking nonsense."

But the little urchin girl whispered to the Queen, "Give her a glass of mead. That will loosen her tongue."

So a jug of mead was brought and the old woman drank one glass, then two, and then said, "Oh, very well. I'll tell you what I know. If you want to have a child you must do exactly as I say. When you go to bed tonight you must wash yourself with two buckets of water. Then throw the water under the bed. When you wake in the morning, look under the bed and you will find two flowers growing. One will be beautiful and one will be ugly. Pick the beautiful one and eat it all. Whatever you do, do not eat the ugly one."

The Queen's face wrinkled in disbelief. "I have never heard such nonsense in my life. Now leave me, all of you!"

She sent the old woman back to the kitchen. In all the commotion the urchin child and her new friend climbed over the palace wall, and straight out of the story!

When the Queen went to bed that night, she thought, "I suppose there would be no harm in trying what that daft old woman suggested."

So the Queen washed herself and threw the water under the bed. When she woke in the morning she peeped underneath. Sure enough, there were two flowers growing! One was beautiful and the other ugly. She was amazed.

The Queen plucked a petal from the beautiful flower and nibbled it. The petal was the most delicious thing she had ever tasted! She quickly ate the flower: leaves, stalk and all! She enjoyed it so much that she began to wonder how the ugly flower would taste. She knew that she should leave it alone, but could not resist slipping a petal into her mouth. What harm could it do? It tasted almost as lovely as the first flower. So she gulped down the whole plant!

Well, the Queen soon dismissed what she had done from her mind, but after a few months her swelling belly reminded her and she realised that she was indeed going to have a baby.

It came time for the babe to be born. In the agony and ecstasy of childbirth, out popped a strange little girl, riding on a white goat and with a wooden spoon thrust before her. The Queen cried out in horror when she saw the little girl, whom she thought very ugly. "Throw a hood over that child's head, for I cannot bear to look at her," croaked the Queen.

An old cloak with a hood was found to cover the child, and so she was named 'Tatterhood'. The little girl rode round and round the room on her goat, shouting, "Don't worry, Mother! There's one much bonnier than me on the way!"

Sure enough, another little girl was born a few minutes later, and the Queen thought her the most beautiful child she had ever seen. She held this infant lovingly in her arms and named her Lily.

You can probably guess which little girl was the Queen's favourite. She made no secret of it either. The Queen wanted nothing to do with Tatterhood and tried to banish her to the Palace kitchens. It was no use however, for wherever Tatterhood was, Lily wanted to be. Lily often felt very sad because of how their mother treated Tatterhood, and would sing to Tatterhood to comfort her:

Now here's to the wee lass, that I love so well,
In style and in beauty no one can excel,
She smiles at me proudly as she sits by my knee,
And there's none in this wide world more happy than me.

Hearing her sister sing made Tatterhood's heart swell. No matter how the Queen treated her, Tatterhood loved Lily, and was always true to herself. She was clever, brave and strong. The girls grew and flourished.

One Christmas Eve, the palace was full of hustle and bustle with preparations. Suddenly the ground began to shake and shudder. Bloodcurdling shrieks rang out in the forest surrounding the palace.

The two girls ran to the Queen and cried, "Mother, Mother! What is happening?"

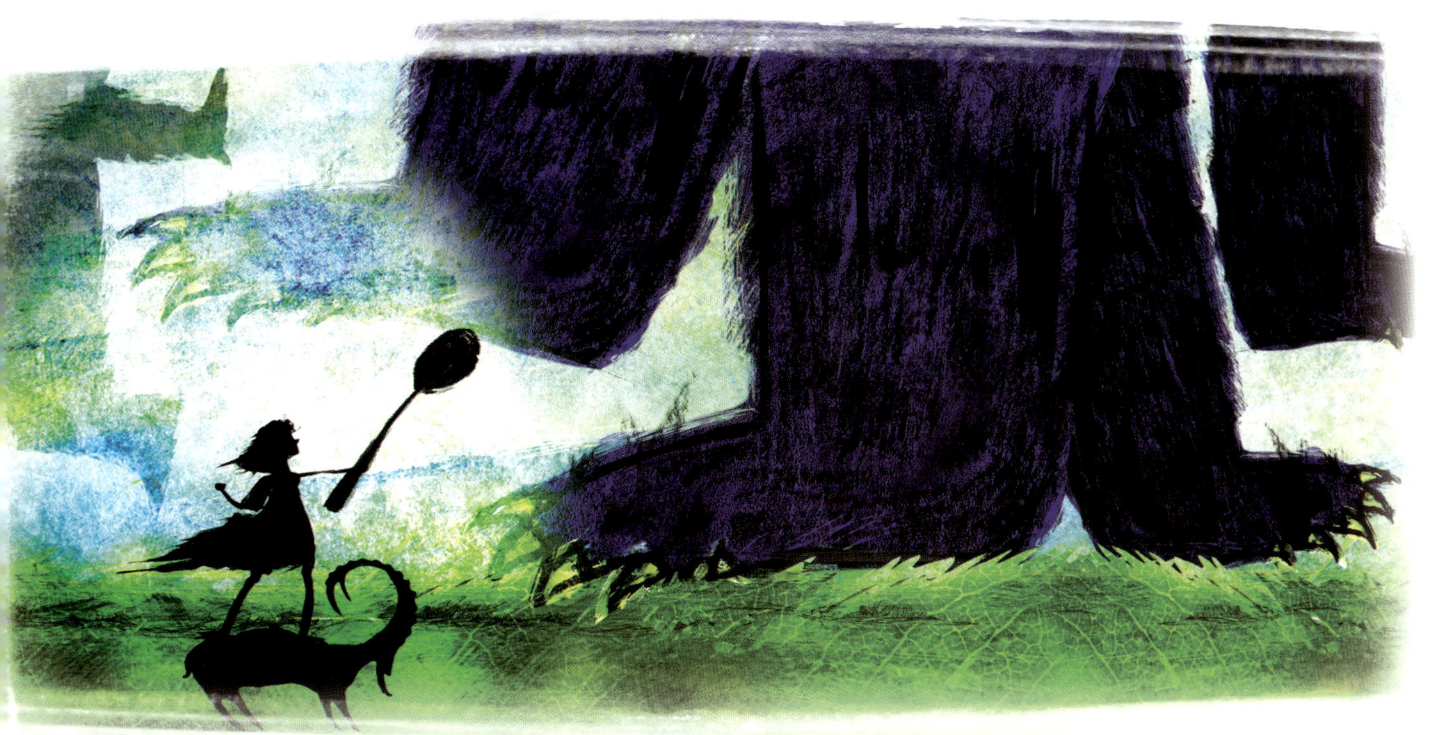

The Queen was pale with fear. "It is the Trolls," she exclaimed, "They have come to steal our Christmas!"

Tatterhood looked at her mother sternly and said, "They will not! I will stop them."

The Queen sneered, "You silly girl, you'll never stop these giant creatures. They will crush you!"

"I am going! Mother, you forget that I have my wooden spoon and my goat! Now promise to keep my sister safe inside and do not open the windows or doors until I return."

So the drawbridge was lowered and Tatterhood trotted out on her goat, her wooden spoon thrust in front of her. Out of the misty forest the enormous Trolls came lumbering towards her, growling. They were huge unsightly creatures, with boils on their faces, and hands that scraped the ground. Tatterhood charged forward on her goat, battering their ankles with her wooden spoon, and soon they were hopping up and down, roaring in agony. Their eyesight was very poor, so they could not see clearly who was causing them such pain. Tatterhood was agile and fast; the Trolls were clumsy and lumbering. Panicked, the Trolls began to retreat into the forest.

Meanwhile, inside the palace, Lily was pacing anxiously up and down, wringing her hands with worry for Tatterhood. Eventually, Lily could stand it no longer and she slowly, carefully, opened the big oak door to peek outside. Instantly, a Troll grabbed Lily's head, twisted it off and put a cow's head in its place!

Having defeated the mighty Trolls, Tatterhood returned in triumph, with her wooden spoon held high. When she saw her sister, she said, "Lily, you opened the door, didn't you?" and in reply Lily could only give a plaintive "Moo!"

Tatterhood then turned to her mother and cried, "Now I will have to pursue the Trolls to get back Lily's pretty head. I need a ship!"

The Queen shook her head disapprovingly but nonetheless provided a ship with a full crew of sailors. Tatterhood declared that she did not need a crew. Rather, she would do all the work by herself.

So Tatterhood set sail with Lily by her side. She manoeuvred the sails, steered the tiller and before long they reached the Land of the Trolls. It was early morning and mist lay over the water like a shroud. Silently Tatterhood dropped anchor and then stood at the widest part of the deck, facing the shore. Then, with her trusty goat and wooden spoon, she trotted as fast as she could towards the ship's edge: trip-trap, trip-trap, trip-trap, whee-eee! Tatterhood flew through the air and landed safely on the shore. There were no Trolls to be seen, so she cantered up the beach until she saw a vast castle. There in a little window at the top of a tall tower was Lily's head! Up the spiral staircase she trotted, and grabbed Lily's head, tucking it under her arm.

As Tatterhood hastened back to the boat, Trolls began to emerge from the sea after their morning bath. They looked huge and frightening. They roared with anger, and lunged clumsily at Tatterhood, who ducked and swerved, clattering their ankles and shins with her spoon. She dodged their gnarled hands skilfully, and at last soared through the air back onto the ship. She raised the anchor swiftly and set sail. The Trolls were left standing on the shore, gazing open-mouthed at their strange opponent, who had beaten them for a second time. When Tatterhood knew they were at a safe distance, she pulled off the cow's head and returned Lily's to its rightful place.

Soon Tatterhood grew tired of sailing, and, reaching a lush green island, decided to stop for a rest. She weighed anchor in a sheltered cove, by a town. Telling Lily to wait below, she merrily trotted around the top deck, chanting, "I am Tatterhood, sailor on the Seven Seas; I am Tatterhood, I sail single-handedly."

The people of the town gathered on the shore, staring at this strange girl wearing a tattered cloak and riding on a goat. They had never seen such a sight!

They shouted to Tatterhood, asking who she was and where she came from. Tatterhood called back commandingly, saying that she would only speak to the ruler of the land.

At last the King approached and Tatterhood agreed that he might come aboard. "So, do you travel alone?" he asked.

"Oh no," replied Tatterhood. "I have my sister Lily with me. She is the most beautiful girl in the world."

"Really?" said the King. "I am looking for a wife, so I'd love to meet her."

Tatterhood agreed and took the King to meet Lily. At first glance he fell in love with Lily and gave her his heart. When he asked Lily to marry him, she answered that since Tatterhood was her elder sister, he should seek her permission in the absence of their mother. Tatterhood smiled at the King's request and said she would agree to the wedding on one condition.

"Well, what is it? Land, jewels, money?" enquired the King.

"Oh no," screeched Tatterhood. "I would like a husband too!"

The King wondered desperately where he could find a match for this strange and wilful girl. At last he resolved to ask his son, the Prince. But how would he persuade him to take on such an unenviable task? He decided to give the Prince a feast of delicate dishes and fine wine. Amazingly, by the end of the evening, the Prince had agreed to the match without having even glimpsed Tatterhood. The wedding was to be the next day!

The streets filled with excited subjects, all eager to see the wedding procession. First came Lily, dressed in a silver and white gown, the finest in the world. She rode upon a chestnut horse and the crowd gasped when they saw her. She really was the most beautiful girl that anyone had seen. The King also looked resplendent in his finery, sitting high upon a dapple-grey horse.

Next came the Prince, handsome in his shining outfit and riding a majestic black horse. He wore a puzzled look on his face and was beginning to regret that he had agreed to this wedding. For by his side trotted Tatterhood, wearing her tattered old cloak, carrying her wooden spoon, and trotting on her white goat. The crowd groaned and murmured as the odd couple passed by. They had never seen such a bride. She had made no effort whatsoever, even on her wedding day!

Tatterhood turned to the Prince and said, "Well, my Prince, now that we have met, do you have any little questions for me before we are married?"

"I certainly do," said the Prince. "For one thing, why do you insist on riding a goat?"

All at once there was a strange tinkling music, and Tatterhood replied, "Why, my Prince, this is a fine white mare! Do you have any other questions?" When the Prince looked again he did indeed see a fine white mare.

"Well, I would also like to know why you always carry that wooden spoon?"

Again the tinkling music could be heard, and Tatterhood replied, "My Prince, this is not a wooden spoon. It is a wand." When the Prince looked again he saw that Tatterhood carried a silver wand, encrusted with precious rubies, sapphires and diamonds.

Finally, he asked, "Why do you wear that tattered old cloak, even on your wedding day?"

"But this is not a cloak," she replied. "This is my wedding dress."

When the Prince looked again, he saw Tatterhood robed most gloriously in a sparkling satin gown.

By the time he reached the altar with Tatterhood, the Prince felt sure that he was looking at the most beautiful girl he had ever seen. But most of all, he had fallen in love with her spirit.

The wedding was a joyous and rowdy affair with much feasting and dancing. The wedding cup was passed around all the guests, and if we hurry there now, we might just catch a last sip . . ..

Follow-on Activity 1

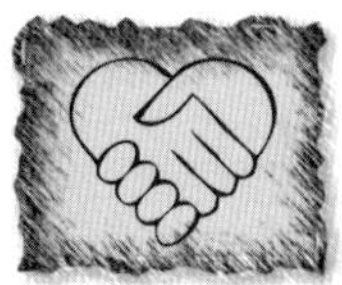

My Hero

In the story, Tatterhood is the hero. Against all odds she rescues her sister's head and then finds happiness and a new life for them both.

We all have heroic qualities inside us. We don't need to have special powers and wear a cloak to be a hero! Nor do we need to perform daring deeds.

This activity, which can be either oral or written, or a mixture of both, asks the children to consider three questions in turn: 'What deeds did Tatterhood perform which made her a hero?'; 'What qualities does Tatterhood have'?; and 'What qualities and actions in your own life might be seen as everyday heroism?'

Aims

- To encourage reflection about ourselves and our positive attributes
- To realise that being a 'hero' is as much about how we lead our lives every day, and about our everyday deeds, as it is about meeting extraordinary challenges
- To emphasise that we can ultimately shape our own destiny: both by being true to ourselves in difficult circumstances, and, when opportunity arises, being ready to move forward

Materials

- Pencil and paper
- Flip chart or whiteboard

Method

The children will be asked to consider three questions in turn:

- What deeds did Tatterhood perform which made her a hero?
- What qualities does Tatterhood have?
- What qualities and actions in your own life might be seen as everyday heroism?

These questions are designed to build towards a realisation that it is Tatterhood's personal qualities rather than just her deeds which make her heroic.

'What deeds did Tatterhood perform which made her a hero?'

Ask the children to discuss this question in pairs, aiming for at least three deeds.
Then bring the group back together.
Write the children's ideas on a flip chart or whiteboard.

'What qualities does Tatterhood have, and how were these shown?'
Again, ask the children to discuss this question in pairs, aiming for at least three examples. There may be a wide variety of responses, such as:

> She is thoughtful: she looks after her sister.
> She is brave: she stands up to her mother, she fights the Trolls, and she asks for what she wants from the King.
> She is resourceful: she can sail a ship without the help of a crew.
> She is unconcerned by the opinion of others: she rides around on a goat and wears a tattered cloak.
> She thinks ahead: she warns Lily not to open the door during the Trolls' attack.
> She is persistent and loyal: she goes to great lengths to get Lily's head back.
> She is clever, and good at planning: she engineers a meeting with the King of the island, and knows what she wants from it.

What qualities and actions in your own life might be seen as everyday heroism?'
The focus in this third stage of the activity shifts from the story to the children's own lives.

A useful bridge is to emphasise that Tatterhood would have possessed all her heroic qualities in daily life, in little deeds, as well as in big adventures. In fact, it is because she would have been like this from day to day that she is able to handle such big challenges.

Ask the children, either in pairs or individually, to consider (and perhaps write down) three 'everyday hero' qualities, with examples of how these have been shown through actions. There may be a wide variety of responses, such as:

> I am strong: yesterday I carried out the recycling box for my Mum.
> I am patient: this morning I waited for my sister while she got ready for school, without getting angry.
> I don't give up: even though I found my maths test hard, I kept trying my best right till the end.

Some children might be more comfortable with a qualifier, such as:

> A few times I have been brave: I once rescued our cat from a tree.
> Sometimes I think ahead: I saved for a present for my Mum's birthday.
> I can be determined: when I lost my favourite hat, I looked everywhere until I found it.

Ask for volunteers to share some of their examples with the wider group.

Follow-on Activity 2

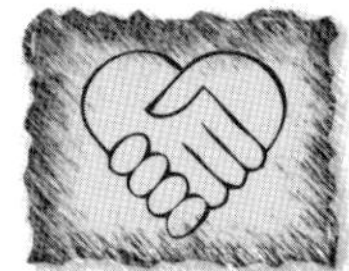

Personal Stories

Stories can lead to other stories, sparked either through imaginative association, or because something in a story resonates with the listener's own experience. Stories can also be handed on, from storyteller to storyteller, and ultimately down the generations. Children may be familiar with this concept, not only from hearing traditional stories, but also, closer to home, from hearing parents' or grandparents' personal stories from when they were young.

This exercise is designed to encourage children to be storytellers themselves. There are two variations in approach.

The first (Method 1) is based around telling an autobiographical anecdote to another, who then re-tells it, second-hand, to a larger group. Done in this way, the exercise illustrates how oral traditions can emerge.

The second (Method 2) allows scope for children to consider and perhaps tell (or write) a story from their own lives, which may be prompted by some element of Tatterhood's tale.

Aims

- To increase confidence in telling oral stories
- To enhance listening skills
- To help children in a group to get to know each other better
- To build relationships by discovering common experiences

Materials

- Just the group!
- Pencil and paper if needed

Method 1:Handing on a story

Ask the children to work in pairs.

Ask them to think of a tale or anecdote, ideally from their own lives, which would take about two minutes to tell.

Explain in advance that the story will first be told to their partner, who will then become the story-teller, re-telling it at second-hand to the larger group. (This helps children to be more concise, and also to listen more carefully.)

The practitioner can decide if the story subject should be left wide open, or guided by a theme, such as:

A treasure which I found . . .
A treasure which I lost . . .
An achievement I felt happy about . . .
An accident I had . . .
A funny thing happened to me . . .
When I was a baby / a toddler . . .
The story of my . . . watch / bicycle / pet / favourite toy

After reflecting for a few minutes, each child then tells their story to their partner.

In the next step, the listener will become the teller. The teller should be encouraged to feel that they now 'own' the story to tell in their own manner, while still being respectful of the original. The originator, who has passed the story on, should be encouraged to let it be re-told without correction. Neither teller nor originator should be overly concerned with fine details (like place names and dates).

When the children are ready to re-tell the story they have heard, gather them together in a circle. (If the group is very large, then circles of six work well).

The teller might introduce the story along the lines:

"This a story of Billy, who once . . ."

After the story-telling, it can be announced that the children are now all fully-fledged storytellers in the oral tradition, having addressed a formal audience!

The stories may subsequently be written up by either the creator, or the re-teller.

Method 2: Linking 'Tatterhood' to a personal story
After listening to 'Tatterhood', children sometimes feel moved to tell a personal story drawn from their own lives. Tatterhood faces many experiences that others can relate to at some time in their lives, such as seeming to be the odd one out, being unpopular with her mother, being comforted by a sibling, confronting bullies, standing up for what she feels is important, and striving for a better life.

Depending on context, the size of the group, and what the practitioner feels is appropriate, children may be invited to tell a story inspired in some way by the story of Tatterhood, based on their own experience.

Sometimes children feel more comfortable telling a story in the third person, even though the story might be based on their own experience: e.g., 'There once was a girl / boy who . . . '.
Because such stories might reflect personal feelings of a sensitive nature, it may be best to confine this activity to pairs, or even for a child to write down the story or outline by themselves, just imagining how it might be told to another person but without actually telling it.

Emphasise to the children that the story they choose to tell or write about should be one that they feel comfortable in sharing.

Follow-on Activity 3

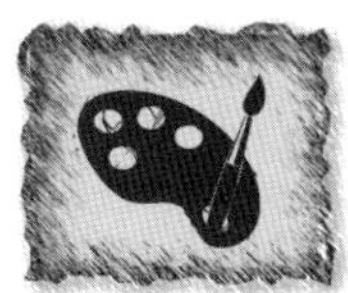

What's Behind the Door?

In the story, Tatterhood tells Lily not to open the front door of the castle while she is away fighting the Trolls. But Lily is anxious for Tatterhood, and cannot bear the suspense of not knowing what is happening. So she opens the door . . ..
This activity invites children to paint an image of a door, and to create a story about what is going on behind it. The door may give clues about what it conceals, or it might have a misleading appearance, or it could be completely neutral.
The children may then tell their 'What's Behind the Door?' story to a group, write it up, or both.

Aims

- To give the imagination free rein, with a sense of 'anything is possible'
- To create a story, with a visual 'peg' either as inspiration or as illustration
- To link conceptual, verbal and artistic imaging
- To promote story-telling and story-listening skills
- Optionally, to translate an oral into a written story

Materials

- Drawing paper
- Paint, or pastels, or coloured pens or pencils

Method

Remind the children of Tatterhood's warning, and of Lily's experience when she opens the door.

Ask the children to make an image of a door, behind which something is happening.

Some children will imagine the door first, and the story second; others will make the door fit their story.

Encourage the children's imaginations to range freely, emphasising that the door may be

- of any material (wood, glass, steel, even marshmallow)
- of any size (ordinary, gigantic, small, microscopic)
- in any building (castle, palace, house, office, school, shop)
- indoors (between rooms; on a cupboard) or outdoors (in a garden, shed or garage)

Invite the children to imagine that they can go through the door and see what is happening behind it. They may go in either direction: from the outside to the inside, or from the inside to the outside.

The style or markings on the door may give hints as to the action beyond or behind it; or may be misleading and belie what is happening; or may be neutral.

After the children have completed their images of a Door, and reflected on what their doors would reveal on being opened, ask the children to take turns to tell their story of 'What is Behind the door'.

The stories may be told either to a partner, or, if the group is small, to the whole group.

The story may subsequently be written up by the teller.

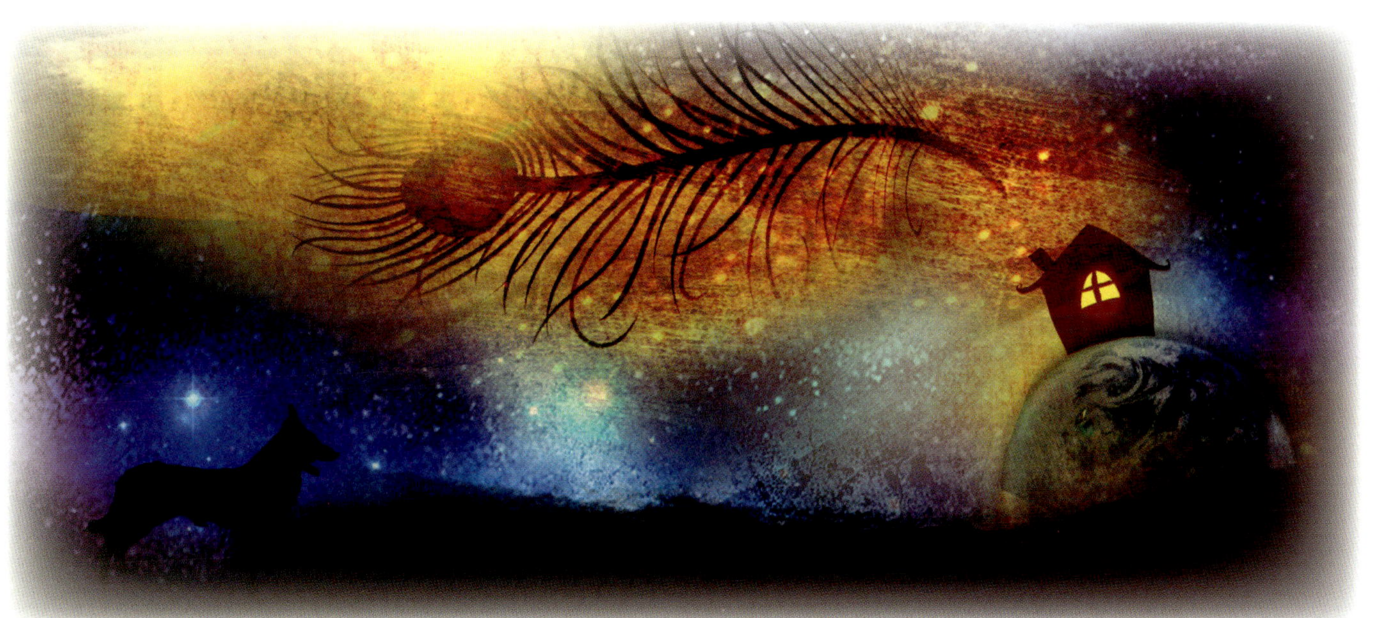

THE DOG AND THE PEACOCK

Introduction

Stage Primary 1 (age 5 years) upwards

Synopsis
A neglected dog and his friends discover that an elderly woman of their village is alone on Christmas Eve. Despite her poverty, she has always been kind and generous. Because of her thoughtfulness towards them during the year, they decide to pay her a surprise visit, bringing their own small offerings. Soon the old woman's cold, dark house is full of warmth and fellowship as she turns their humble presents into a modest feast. The friends also make a special Christmas decoration as a gift, which greatly moves the old woman. They enjoy a happy party together.

Background
This touching story hails from Scotland, and while set at Christmas, has a universal message. It emphasises the importance of repaying kindness with kindness, and the importance of considering those who are not so well off, especially at festive times. There is a message, too, about the nature of gifts. In 'The Dog and the Peacock', the most splendid gift to the old woman is the creatures' presence – just 'being there'. It is welcome relief from the materialism which can prevail at Christmastime.

Suggested Themes

- Thinking about others less fortunate than ourselves, especially older people
- Repaying kind deeds with kindness
- Minimising the need for material gifts in life
- Challenging the consumerism of modern-day Christmas
- How thinking creatively, and working as a team, can lead to good results

Skeleton

1. An old collie lives on the street, having been replaced on the farm by a younger dog.
2. He notices that the house of a kind old woman looks dark and cold, when all other homes are bright and merry. There is no fire lit or candles glowing in the old woman's house.
3. The Dog visits his friend, the Peacock, who reveals that it is Christmas Eve.
4. The Dog asks the Peacock if his master might spare some peat to give to the old woman for her fireplace, in return for her kindness in giving them scraps of food throughout the year.
5. Carrying a brick of peat under each wing, the Peacock sets off with the Dog to visit the old woman.
6. They are joined by the Cat, who, learning of their destination, fetches some kippers from the fishmonger's shop.
7. The Dog, following the Cat's example, then finds some discarded sausages at the butcher's.
8. When they reach the old woman's house, their friend the Owl asks if he may join them, although he has no gift to bring.
9. The old woman answers their knock on the door, saying sadly that she has no food to offer them.
10. But the visitors slip past her into the house, and give her their presents.
11. The old woman is very touched. She goes to cook the food while her visitors light the fire.
12. The Owl then has an idea for another gift. He shares his idea with the other creatures.
13. When the old woman returns to the sitting room, she sees the most beautiful Christmas decoration ever: the Cat and the Owl sit on each side of the hearth, their eyes reflecting the firelight; and between them, lit from behind, the Peacock displays his splendid feathers.
14. The friends share food, stories and company, on a Christmas Eve that they will all remember as special.

THE DOG AND THE PEACOCK

The old sheepdog trotted through the cold, empty streets. His head low, he was looking for any scraps of food he could find. He had been a good working dog, but had grown slow with age. So his master, a farmer, had replaced him with a new collie. The old dog found himself on the street, all alone. The only human to show him kindness was a poor old woman who lived by herself.

Snow began to fall and the Dog looked sadly into the houses filled with people, candlelight and merriment. When he came to the old woman's house he saw that it was dark, without even a plume of smoke coming from the chimney. "Strange," thought the Dog. "The old lady can usually be counted on for a pat and a few scraps. I hope all is well with her."

In fact, the whole town seemed deserted, with everyone indoors. The Dog was puzzled. At the end of the street he saw a peacock perched on the gatepost of the Big House.

"Evening, Collie," shouted the Peacock. "What are you up to this Christmas Eve?"

"Christmas Eve! So that's why the street is so quiet. Well, I am a bit worried about the old woman. Her house is in darkness. Do you think your master would miss a few bricks of peat? I could take them as a Christmas gift. Then she would at least have a fire."

"Of course he wouldn't mind. He has a houseful of party guests and my wife is busy sitting on an egg, so I can come with you."

The Peacock placed a brick of peat under each wing, and set off with the Dog through the deserted streets. It wasn't long before a ginger cat leapt over a wall.

"Where are you two going?" yowled the Cat.

"We're off to see the old woman with some peat for her fire. She's so good to us all year round. But we think she's alone in the darkness on Christmas Eve," said the Dog.

"Well, I know a way into the fishmonger's shop. I could fetch a few kippers. I'm sure he wouldn't mind, being for the old woman after all."

So the Cat slipped through the back window of the fishmonger's and brought out a pair of kippers in her mouth. Then the Dog had an idea. He knew that the butcher would have left any sausages he hadn't sold behind his shop. He disappeared and soon returned with a string of pork sausages.

"We'll give the old woman a Christmas Eve to remember!" exclaimed the Dog, as the three pals trotted down the street together.

At last they reached the old woman's house, and there on the gate sat an owl.

"Hoo hoo! What are you lot up to?" asked the Owl.

"We're visiting the old woman, bringing fuel for her fire and food for her table. She is so good to us all year round, and we thought we'd return a little of her kindness," said the Peacock.

"Hoo hoo, great idea! I'd like to come too, although I have nothing to bring," hooted the Owl.

"Come along," cried the friends. "The more the merrier!"

They approached the dark door and knocked as loudly as their paws, wings and beaks would let them. As they waited, the Owl whispered, "I have an idea for what else we can give. I'll show you inside."

The old woman eventually opened the door and smiled gently when she saw her unexpected visitors. Sadly she declared, "I'm sorry my friends, but I have no food for you tonight."

The creatures slipped past the old woman and into her house. She was touched when she saw their gifts, and asked them to light the fire while she cooked the food. Soon there was a warm glow in the fireplace and a smell of kippers in the air. The Owl whispered his idea to his fellows.

When the old woman returned with the feast, she gasped with surprise and delight. The Cat was sitting on one side of the hearth and the Owl on the other, their eyes reflecting the flickering firelight. Between them, the Peacock stood with his splendid tail feathers fanned out, shimmering in the orange light.

"That is the most wonderful Christmas decoration I have ever seen," exclaimed the old woman joyfully.

The friends sat together and shared the feast. They told stories, sang songs, and laughed at jokes. Truly, it was a Christmas Eve to remember.

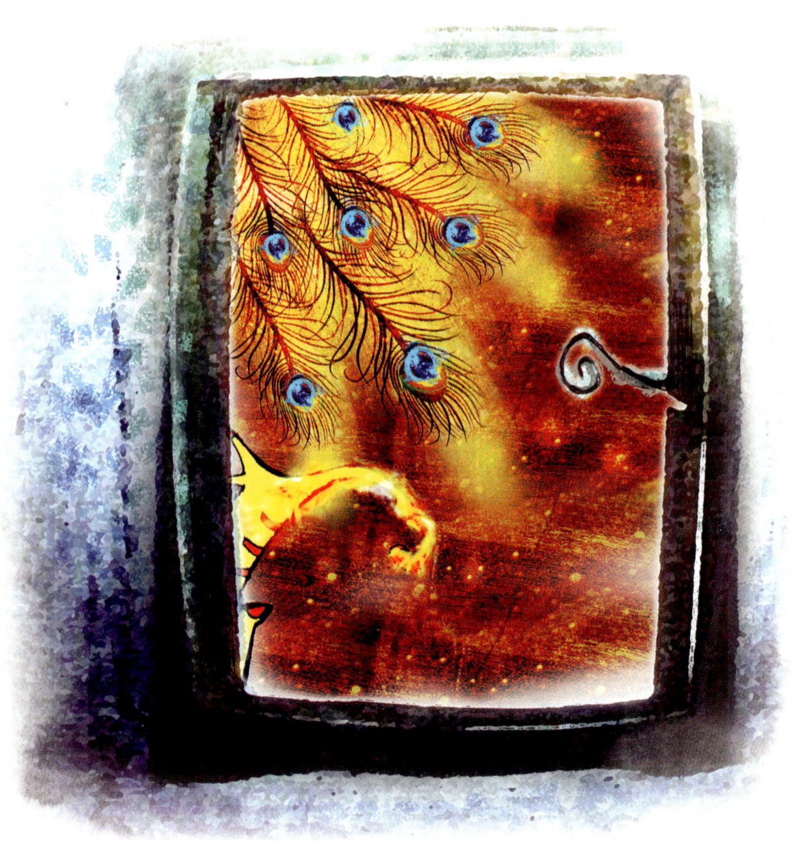

Follow-up Activity 1

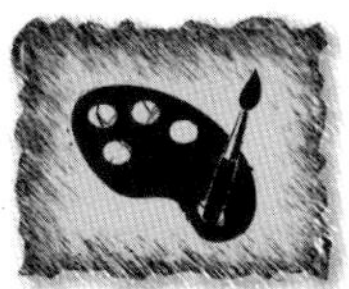

Customise a Candle

In the story, the glowing fire is an image of warmth and togetherness. It also lights up the Christmas decoration which the friends make for the old woman, illuminating their best gift of all: being there.

In this activity, the children decorate a plain candle with pieces of coloured beeswax, making a personalised candle. The candles may be planned as a gift. Alternatively, the individually-decorated candles may be used as part of a group exercise.

'Customise a Candle' as a group-based exercise can be very effective at the beginning of a group programme, or at the beginning of term. In the first session, each child decorates their own candle. Then each week the children can 'arrive' in the group by lighting their candle and taking turns to say a few words about how they feel about being in the group on that day. This creates a reassuring verbal and visual ritual, and encourages fellowship. It also acknowledges and illustrates that each child is individual and different, yet a part of the group.

The candles can provide a glow while the story 'The Dog and the Peacock' (or indeed, any other story) is told, reminiscent of a traditional fireside.

Note: Permission may be needed before using lighted candles. If these are not permitted, battery-operated (electric) tealights or candles can be substituted. Some of these are made of real wax, and so may be decorated as outlined below. If real candles are used, they may cause great excitement at first, especially if candles are a new experience. The children may initially need some boundaries around the presence of the candles in order to stay safe. It can be worth persevering with children's exuberance or fear until they enjoy the atmosphere of peace that candlelight can bring. A taper for lighting, and a candle-snuffer for extinguishing, should be used.

Aims

These may include:

- Creating a sense of belonging within a group
- Encouraging expression of individualism within group
- Giving a sense of reassurance by having the same beginning ritual for each session
- Conveying a traditional atmosphere for telling the story
- Marking a festive occasion, such as Christmas
- Making a gift, or a memento

Materials

- Plain candles, preferably beeswax (pillar-shaped gives a large area to decorate), **or**
- Battery-operated wax candles (preferably pillar-shaped)
- Sheets of coloured beeswax for decorating (Stockmar Modelling Beeswax, from craft stockists; or from Salago.co.uk or Amazon.co.uk)
- A blunt-edged knife, such as a butter knife, and chopping board or plate
- Taper for lighting, and candle-snuffer for extinguishing candles

Method

Decide whether the candles are to be gifts, or to be used in a series of group-based sessions, or as a backdrop for storytelling (or a combination of these).

Demonstrate how to decorate a candle (or have a pre-prepared example):

1. From the wax sheets, cut small pieces of wax with a blunt knife.
2. Point out that simple geometric shapes such as triangles or squares are easier than intricate or curved shapes. Thin strips also work well.
3. Rub each piece of wax gently onto the surface of the candle. Warmed by the heat of a hand, wax will stick to the candle, as if by magic.

To ensure that each child has enough decorating wax, and that popular colours are distributed fairly, sheets may be pre-cut and handed out.

Follow-on Activity 2

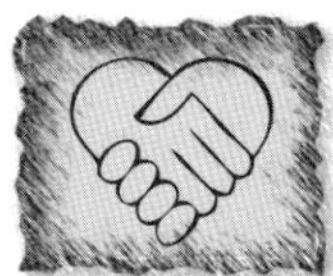

Let's have a Ceilidh!

In this story, the friends have a Christmas Eve to remember, by coming together and sharing stories, songs, jokes and food. In Scotland such a gathering is called a 'ceilidh' (pronounced *kay-lee*), but in all cultures this is how people spent time together before the days of radio, television or computer games.

There is an old saying, 'The fire burns brightest if we each add a piece of wood.'. In this activity, the children hold their own ceilidh, each child being encouraged to contribute something individually, in pairs, or in small groups. They may recite a poem; tell a story, joke or riddle; sing a song; play an instrument; or perform or teach a dance.

Aims

- To help children to get to know each other
- To develop skills in listening and talking
- To build self-esteem and self-confidence
- To teach children that entertainment can be active and participatory

Materials

- The children's own preparation, either individually, in pairs or in small groups. (See next, under Method.)
- For the practitioner's use, a running order with an approximation of timings.

Method

Introduce the concept of a ceilidh to the children.

Give examples of the kinds of contributions they might like to make to their own ceilidh. These might include

- A poem
- A story (such as stories from this pack, told or acted out by pairs or small groups; or an anecdote, perhaps drawing on a funny or poignant family story: 'When my granny was a girl . . ., etc.')
- A joke (or several)
- A riddle (These are popular, and are usually short enough to recite. Books or the Internet are a good source. See 'Presenting Riddles', below.)
- A song (See 'Presenting Songs', below)
- A tune played on an instrument
- A dance, either performed, or taught (i.e., with everyone joining in)

Ask the children to let you know in advance what they want to do, so that a mixed programme can be prepared. Work out the time allowance for each item, so that everyone will have a chance to present their 'turn'. In a large group, the ceilidh may need to be held in several parts.

Encourage the children to prepare or rehearse in advance, but aim for an atmosphere of ‘sharing’ rather than ‘performing’, so that the activity is fun rather than an ordeal. Even with a programme outlined, and approximate times allocated, it is important to keep a sense of informality and spontaneity if possible.

While some children may be shy at first, ceilidhs tend to build up momentum as more and more children pile in with jokes, riddles and on-the-spot performances. Some tips for presentation and participation follow.

Presenting Riddles
If a child presents a riddle, ask for the riddle question to be repeated several times. Then, to maximise participation, invite the other children to join in, reciting the riddle question together. Encourage the children to raise their hands if they want to give an answer. Let the child who has brought the riddle select a child to have a guess. (Nb: this procedure can be worked out in advance with those children presenting riddles.)

Presenting Songs
Find out in advance if a child wants to present a solo, or have everyone sing a chorus, or sing solo and then have everyone join in a second time round. If it is a less well-known song, printing and distributing the words might help.

Presenting Stories
If encouraging a group of children to tell a story, ‘The Cockerel and the Sultan’ is ideal. Using the Story Skeleton as a guide, the story may be divided into up to six parts, with each child standing in line and telling a section.

All contributions to the ceilidh, however small, should be celebrated with a round of applause, and with positive feedback from the practitioner.

Follow-on Activity 3

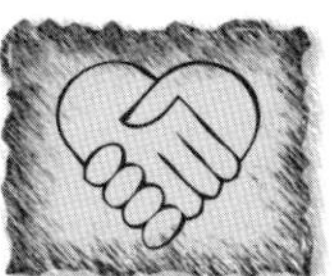

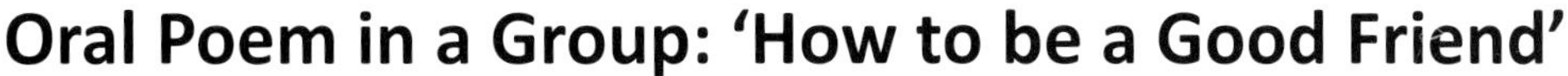

Oral Poem in a Group: 'How to be a Good Friend'

In the story 'The Dog and the Peacock', the Dog, the Peacock, the Cat and the Owl thought about an old woman being alone and then acted as good friends to her.

In this exercise, the whole group makes an oral poem based on the theme of friendship. The children are each asked to contribute a line about being a friend, and after each line the group choruses the refrain, 'How to be a Good Friend'.

This activity is a version of 'The Good Goodbye, Follow-on Activity 2, Oral Poem: "The Things We Remember from Primary School"'.

Aims

- To build cohesion in the group
- To encourage reflection about the meaning of friendship
- To bring ideas together in a creative way

Materials

- The group, seated in a circle
- Thumb piano, lyre or other quiet instrument

Method

The children should be seated in a circle. Ask them each to think, in one sentence, of something that they can do, or have done, to be a good friend.

Ideas might include:

> Giving flowers to cheer someone up
> Noticing that someone is alone in the playground
> Inviting someone to play a game
> Sharing sweets
> Singing a song together
> Laughing together
> Telling jokes together
> Asking if someone is ok when they look sad
> Asking about someone's new hobby

Go around the circle asking for each child's sentence in turn. Between each contribution the refrain 'How to be a good friend' is repeated by the whole group.

Sometimes, hearing other ideas may spark a new train of thought, so that children may ask to revise their contribution.

When the children are happy with their choices, ask them to fit their sentence into a specified number of words (such as six words, or eight), so that everyone's line is the same length. (They may need to add or take away a few words, rendering their thought as a poetic phrase rather than as a grammatical sentence.)

Go around the group again, with each child saying their own line in turn, interspersed with the refrain from everyone. A steady rhythm will emerge.

Once the children feel confident with their words, music may be added. A thumb piano or lyre works well as background accompaniment. The child preceding the speaker is given the instrument and while one child speaks, the other plays a little tune. The instrument is then passed to the next child, while the refrain is spoken by everyone. This sequence is repeated around the circle.

Children tend to be patient and respectful with each other in this activity, and are keen to hear what lines their peers will add to the poem.

The end result is a wonderful rhythmic poem, chant or song that leaves children with a sense of wonder and accomplishment, as well as something which helps process their thoughts about friendship.

It can be useful to make an audio recording of the final version of the poem; copies might even be made as a souvenir.

Alternatively, the poem can be written down by a scribe and either hung on the wall for the children to feel proud of, or photocopied for the children to keep.

THE GOOD GOODBYE

Introduction

Stage Primary 5 (age 9) upwards

Synopsis
A teacher is trying to find a suitable way to farewell her Primary 7 class. She tells the children of a dream in which she visited another planet. All the people of this planet wear grey cloaks throughout their lives. When a person dies, a 'Goodbye Ceremony' is held, during which the 'story' of that person's life is told through the emerging colours and decorations on the cloak.

Background
This story was indeed inspired by a dream similar to that depicted here. It is very valuable for Primary 7 transition work before high school. However, it can also be used more generally to encourage children to reflect on what they consider to be the most important values, what kind of person they wish to be, what they have done with their lives so far, and what they hope to achieve in the future.

Suggested Themes

- The values which we choose to live by
- The importance of saying goodbye
- The significance of endings and new beginnings, and of transition points in life
- The meaningful nature of the teacher-pupil relationship

Skeleton

1. A teacher is retiring, and the children whom she has taught for many years are preparing for high school. She wishes to give them a special gift to say goodbye.
2. While asleep, a vivid dream comes to her. This inspires a story which becomes her gift.
3. The next day she takes her class out for a special lunch, and tells them of her dream.
4. She dreamt that she visited another planet where everyone is clad in a grey cloak.
5. She finds herself part of a large crowd, attending an old man's funeral.
6. A young boy explains that this is a 'Goodbye' ceremony. As she watches, the elderly man's grey cloak is transformed.
7. The boy explains further that during the Goodbye ceremony, a person's cloak takes on colours and patterns which tell the true story of the life which has been led: of the person's qualities, values and deeds. Some lives are shown in beautiful, vivid cloaks, others in faded, tattered ones.
8. The teacher tells the children that she recognised their faces in the crowd of her dream, and that if she had such a cloak, it would surely show their time together.
9. Her last wish is that they live life well and fully, so that their cloaks will be splendid.

THE GOOD GOODBYE

Mrs Maltman was tired. Tomorrow would be the last day of term and her Primary 7 class would leave for a new chapter of life in high school. She could remember their shining little faces on their first day of school! But it was not just the children who would leave Killowen Primary for the last time tomorrow, for it would also be Mrs Maltman's last day of teaching after thirty years in the same school.

That evening she went to bed early, gently closed her eyes, and thought of the children in her class. "I would dearly love to give them a gift," she thought, "something special that they can take with them when they leave me".

She drifted off to sleep and began to dream. When she awoke it was morning. Remembering her dream she smiled, thinking, 'Now I have the perfect gift for the children.'

When Mrs Maltman arrived at school that morning she gathered her class around her and said, "Children this is a very important day for you. It is your last day at primary school, and so I have planned something special for you all. I want you to put on your coats and follow me down to the village."

So the children all filed out of the school after her, wondering where they were going. When they reached the hotel on Main Street, Mrs Maltman led them to a room upstairs. There a table was spread with a beautiful cloth and Mrs Maltman had written each of their names in calligraphy on an individual place-card.

The children took their seats and they were served a delicious feast. Then Mrs Maltman asked them all to be quiet. She began to tell a story . . .

"Last night, I dreamt that I travelled in a spaceship to a land faraway. When I landed there I was swept up in a huge crowd of people who were all walking in the same direction. I noticed that everyone was dressed in the same plain grey cloaks which smelt sweet as wildflowers.

"After a while we came to a great town square and the people stopped. There, raised up on a stone plinth lay the body of an old man. He seemed dead but his body was wrapped in the same grey cloak as the others.

"The crowd began to chant, 'God bless you . . . Goodbye . . . Goodbye, and Hello'.

"I was confused, so I asked a young boy beside me, 'What is happening?'

"'Don't you know? We are celebrating this man's life - it is a ceremony of goodbye,' he explained.

"'But why do the people also chant, "Hello"?' I enquired.

"'Well,' he began, 'because every "Goodbye" is also a "Hello".'

"Then something amazing happened, for the most beautiful shapes, patterns and iridescent colours began to appear on the man's cloak. It was as if invisible hands were weaving these wonderful designs in red, blue and gold.

"'What does this mean?' I asked the boy by my side.

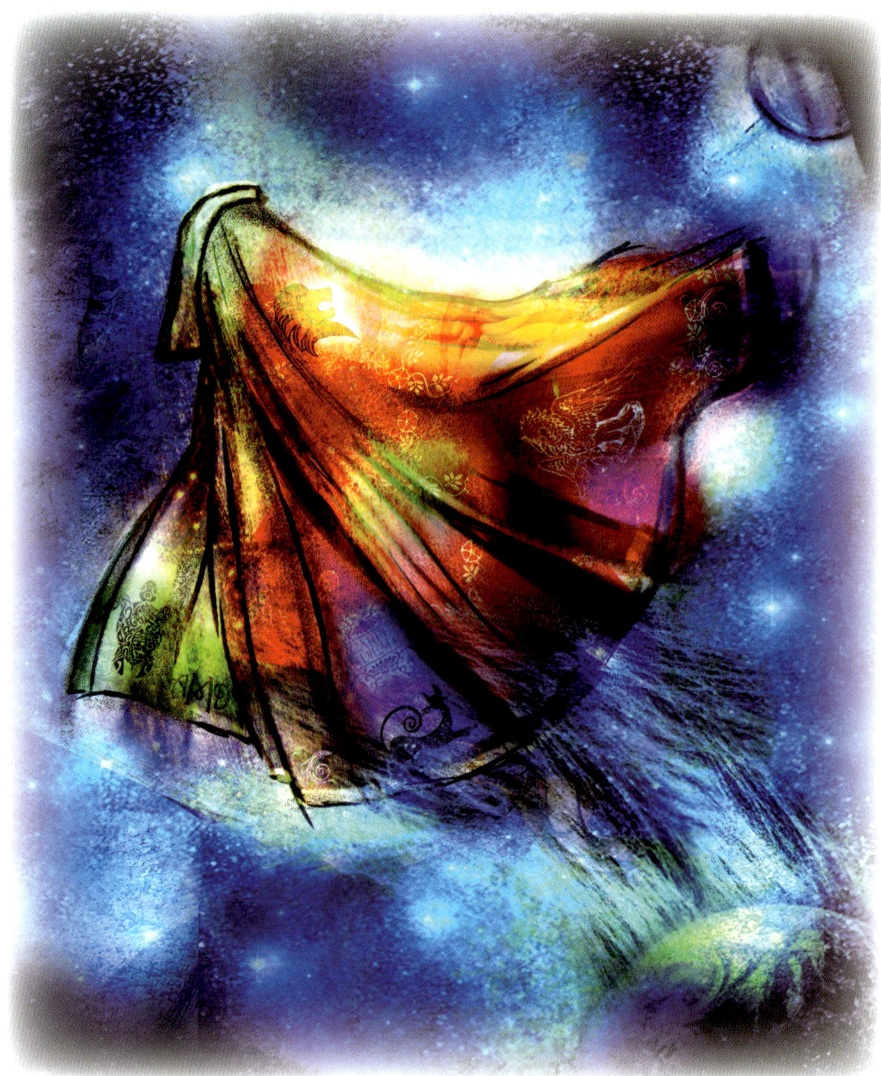

"'The colours and shapes you see on the man's cloak tell the story of his life,' said the boy. 'The blue shows he was loyal, the red that he had a courageous heart, and the gold that he was loving to others.'

"Feeling curious, I asked, 'Is everyone's cloak as beautiful as this?'

"'No,' explained the boy, 'This was a good man, he led a good life. But when some people reach the end of their life, their cloak just frays, tatters and turns to dust. For others there are only faint patches of colour. The cloak will reflect the kind of life which that person has led.'

"Well, the next thing I remember, I woke up with the golden light of morning streaming through my window. When I recalled my dream, I thought that some of the people I had seen in the crowd were familiar to me, and then I laughed because I realised that I had seen all of you in the crowd."

Then she gazed intently at the children with a misty look in her eyes and continued, "Children, you are all young and your stories are just beginning. I can tell you that if I had a cloak at the end of my life, our time together would be represented there. My hope for you is that you will live your lives gloriously, so that the 'Goodbye Cloaks' of your life will be splendid to behold."

Follow-on Activity 1

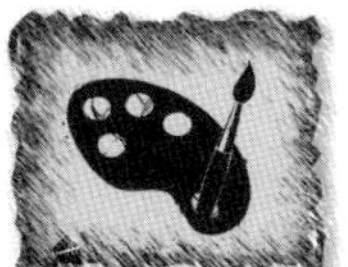

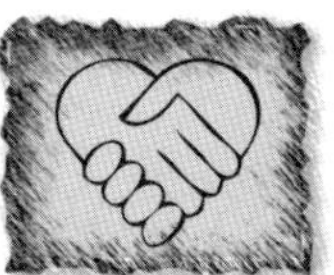

Design a Cloak

This activity, in which children each draw and colour a cloak which represents aspects of their own lives, is designed to encourage reflection and mindfulness.

Aims

- To encourage the children to reflect on their own values in life
- To help the children consider that their actions in life are noticed by their community and do matter to others
- To consider how we would like to be seen by others

Materials

- Felt pens, coloured pencils
- Paper with a 'cloak' outline already drawn (it saves time to have this photocopied in advance)

Method

Invite the children to think about how the old man's cloak told the story of his life, and how its colours and images represented the things he had done, and the qualities he had as a person: "The blue shows he was loyal, the red that he had a courageous heart and the gold that he was loving."

Encourage the children to reflect on what qualities, experiences and deeds they would include on their own cloak at this point in their lives. Some children might benefit from a discussion as to what areas this may cover e.g. thinking of others, being a good friend, a loving sister or brother, or a reliable team-member; being honest, optimistic, funny or cheerful; trying hard in maths, persevering in spelling, or keeping their desks tidy; etc., etc.

This exercise may raise negative as well as positive reflections from the children; the practitioner may need to use discretion in how this is managed.

Ask each child to fill in their own cloak, representing their lives so far. This might include images but perhaps just colour and patterns.

A key at the side of the picture can explain what the different colours and images represent.

Ask volunteers to describe their finished cloaks to the rest of the group.

Ask the children if, as a result of this exercise, their outlook or aspirations have been affected.

When they have completed the cloak, they can be asked to share their picture with the rest of the group.

Follow-on Activity 2

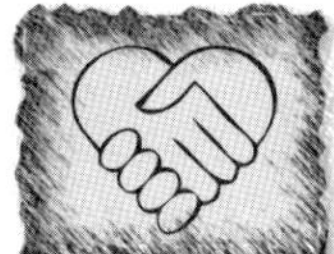

Oral Poem in a Group: 'The Things We Remember from Primary School'

In this exercise the whole group makes an oral poem after identifying a subject, and agreeing a shared refrain such as 'The things we remember from primary school', or 'Our hopes and fears for high school', or 'The best things about the holidays'.

This activity can be adapted to many circumstances. It can be particularly useful for children passing from primary to secondary school, which is the theme of 'The Good Goodbye'. It provides an occasion either to look back (farewelling primary school), or forward (anticipating high school).

While this exercise can help children to look forward in a positive manner, it may also raise issues that can usefully be addressed in preparing for high school.

Aims
- To build cohesion in the group
- To encourage reflection
- To acknowledge loss and change in a creative way

Materials
- The group, seated in a circle
- Thumb piano, lyre or other quiet instrument

Method
The children should be seated in a circle. Ask them each to think, in one sentence, of something that they will always remember from their days at primary school. It might relate to a memorable event, or significant emotion; or it might reflect everyday life. If anyone has difficulty, suggest that they consider their senses: what have they seen, heard, smelt, tasted, or touched.

Go around the circle asking for each child's sentence in turn. Between each contribution the refrain 'The things we remember from primary school' is repeated by the whole group.

Sometimes, hearing other memories may spark a new train of thought, so that children may ask to revise their contribution.

When the children are happy with their choices, ask them to fit their memory into six words, so that everyone's line is the same length. (They may need to add or take away a few words, rendering their memory as a poetic phrase rather than as a grammatical sentence.)

Go around the group again, with each child saying their own six-word line in turn, interspersed with the refrain from everyone. A steady rhythm will emerge.

Once the children feel confident with their words, music may be added. A thumb piano or lyre works well as background accompaniment. The child preceding the speaker is given the instrument and while one child speaks, the other plays a little tune. The instrument is then passed to the next child, while the refrain is spoken by everyone. This sequence is repeated around the circle.

Children tend to be patient and respectful with each other in this activity, and are keen to hear what memories others will add.

The end result is a wonderful rhythmic poem, chant or song that leaves children with a sense of wonder and accomplishment, as well as something which helps process their experiences.

It can be useful to make an audio recording of the final version of the poem; copies might even be made as a souvenir.

Alternatively the poem can be written down by a scribe and either hung on the wall for the children to feel proud of, or photocopied for the children to keep.

Follow on Activity 3

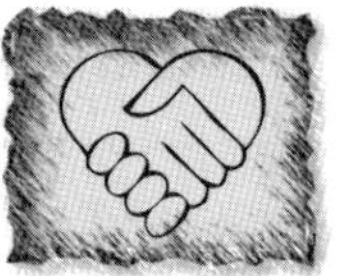

Give a Blessing

This story, and this activity, are effective when used in a final session with a group (or an individual) being farewelled, or entering a new phase of life.

Blessings were used traditionally in many cultures and were considered very precious. There are many different types of blessing. Some may celebrate individual qualities, while others may wish general good fortune. As in 'The Seven Ravens', blessings were often given to people setting out on a journey. It was hoped that the blessing would give the traveller protection and good luck. Blessings were also often given at the beginning of a new stage in life's journey: at birth, at passage to adolescence or adulthood, at marriage, or on other significant occasions. In 'The Good Goodbye', the children in Mrs Maltman's class are on the verge of a new chapter of life.

The natural world can inspire many different images, similes and metaphors, and is often the basis for traditional blessings.

This activity, in which blessings are composed, delivered and received, can be used effectively at times of transition or ending. Many children find such times challenging, leading to emotional or behavioural issues. Ceremony and ritual can alleviate the negative aspects of an ending, making it meaningful and positive.

Aims

- To promote a feeling of shared experience in the group
- To value each person's unique qualities
- To provide a positive experience of a transition or an ending
- To show how powerful and precious words can be
- To introduce the practice of thinking carefully about the words, and of composing and drafting before writing out a final version.

Materials

- Scrap paper to draft blessings on
- Card, ribbon and coloured writing pens
- Optional: flowers and candles (**note**: permission might be needed for the latter; if allowed, a taper and candle-snuffer are useful)

Method

Explain the background to blessings, and possible occasions for their use.

As an example, re-visit the blessing from 'The Seven Ravens' story: "May the love in your heart give you the strength to travel with the bravery of a lioness, the surefootedness of a donkey and the shrewdness of a fox." Further examples are given below.

For this activity, blessings may either be composed by the practitioner for individual children, or by the children for each other.

It is a good idea to do a first draft on scrap paper and then a fair copy on card.

Once written in their final form, a ceremony can be held to exchange blessings.

More detail about composing and presenting blessings follows:

Blessings composed by the practitioner

At the end of a period of contact, the practitioner can write a blessing for each child. It can be an appropriate and powerful gift: heartfelt, affirming and unique to each child. The practitioner may know the subject well and be able to highlight their particular qualities and strengths in the blessing. However, if this is not the case, then this exercise can be preceded by the 'What are You Best at in the World?' exercise ('Finn McCool', Follow-on Activity 3).

Here are two examples. For Bob, who says he is good at building,

> *May you build your life on a strong foundation, on rock and not sand.*
> *May you have the wisdom of the third little pig, who built her house out of bricks, not straw or sticks.*
> *May the big bad wolves flee into the forest when they are met with your fearlessness and quick wits.*

For Rebecca, who says she is good at art,

> *May your paint palette always be full of all the colours of the rainbow.*
> *May you learn to paint life in all its vibrant colours.*
> *May you discover the sunshine and the rainbows which always follow the rain.*

Blessings composed by the child

Alternatively, children may write a blessing for each other. Names can be drawn from a hat in order to decide who writes for whom. It may be helpful to provide an example from a traditional source, such as this old Celtic blessing.

> *May the road rise up to meet you,*
> *May the wind always be at your back,*
> *May the sun shine warm upon your face,*
> *May the rain fall soft upon your field,*
> *And until we meet again,*
> *May God hold you in the palm of his hand.*

For children needing more structure, a template may be given.

> *May you have the* _____ [quality] *of* _____ [a time of day],
> *May you have the* _____ [quality] *of* _____ [a place in nature],
> *May you have the* _____ [quality] *of* _____ [type of weather],
> *And may you always have the* _____ [quality] *of* ______ [an animal or bird].

Presentation of blessings
Once the blessings have been composed on scrap paper they can be carefully copied either directly onto a piece of coloured card, or else onto a decorated piece of paper, perhaps using coloured pens. It can be extra special to write the verse on a piece of paper and then insert it into a decorated folded card, fixing it with a ribbon.

A ceremony can be held to give out the blessings. The room can be decorated with flowers, and perhaps a candle lit for each person. As each name is called, the author of a blessing then reads it aloud for that person. The card is handed over, hands are shaken and then the receiver extinguishes his or her candle. This continues until each person has been given their blessing. This process can be moving, and engages children deeply if done in a reverential and special way.

SOURCES

I give thanks and acknowledgement to the following for inspiration, and encourage users of this pack to explore these sources further.

SOURCES FOR STORIES

'The Legend of Beira and Bride'
Co-written with Claire McNicol. See also Donald Alexander Mackenzie, *Wonder Tales from Scottish Myth and Legend*, London, Blackie and Son, 1917.

'The Taen Awa'
Told to me by Steven Walker of the Craigmillar Children's Project Storytelling Group, run by Claire McNicol. Inspired by Duncan Williamson's *The Broonie, Silkies and Fairies*, Edinburgh, Canongate, 1985.

'The Seven Ravens'
Originally collected from German storytellers in the early nineteenth century by the Brothers Grimm, and included in many *Grimm's Fairy Tales* compilations since. For instance Jacob and Wilhelm Grimm, *Grimms' Fairy Tales*, London, Puffin Books, 1994.

'Finn McCool and the Young Hero's Children'
Told to me by Fergus McNicol and co-written with Claire McNicol. For more tales of Finn, see Rosemary Sutcliff, *The High Deeds of Finn MacCool*, London, Red Fox, 2001.

'One-Eye, Two-Eyes, Three-Eyes'
Inspired by the telling of renowned traveller Betsy Whyte. Recording held by Tobar an Dualchais (Kist o' Riches), an on-line archive (www.tobarandualchais.co.uk) of Gaelic and Scots oral recordings from the School of Scottish Studies (University of Edinburgh), BBC Scotland and National Trust for Scotland.

'The Cockerel and the Sultan'
Told to me by my daughter, Sylva, after her teacher Lucila Mucado's telling at The Edinburgh Steiner School.

'Tatterhood'
Inspired by the telling of Claire McNicol.

'Jack and Marigold'
Inspired by the telling of Stanley Robertson. Recording held by Tobar an Dualchais (Kist o' Riches), an on-line archive (www.tobarandualchais.co.uk) of Gaelic and Scots oral recordings from the School of Scottish Studies (University of Edinburgh), BBC Scotland and National Trust for Scotland. My thanks to Robbie Robertson for permission. See also Stanley Robertson, *Exodus to Alford,* Edinburgh, Balnain Books, 1988.

'The Dog and the Peacock'
Told to me by Claire McNicol. After Duncan Williamson, *Tell Me a Story for Christmas*, Edinburgh, Canongate, 1987 and currently in Duncan Williamson, *Land of the Seal People*, Edinburgh, Birlinn, 2010.

'The Good Goodbye'
Inspired by 'The Goodbye Cloak', in David Campbell, *Tales to Tell II*, Edinburgh, Saint Andrew Press, 1994. David wrote this story after being told a dream by a woman whom he met on a bus journey in the Middle East.

SOURCES FOR ACTIVITIES
Many of the activities were inspired by others:
'Give a Blessing': developed in collaboration with Claire McNicol
'Make a Creation Myth': Claire McNicol
'Oral Poem in a Group': adapted from Helen East (www.eastorywilsound.co.uk)
'Harvesting a Story': Fergus McNicol (www.macastory.co.uk)
'Story Map': Fergus McNicol
'Arruchica': Fergus McNicol
'Envelope Puppets': Linda McCann (canndhu.com)
'Story Sticks': Wendy Dacre (www.raventales.co.uk)

INTRODUCTION: SECONDARY SOURCES
Bettelheim, Bruno, *The Uses of Enchantment: The Meaning and Importance of Fairy Tales*, New York, Knopf, 1976.

Gerhardt, Sue, *Why Love Matters: How Affection Shapes a Baby's Brain,* Hove, Routledge, 2004.

OTHER RESOURCES FOR STORYTELLERS

The Scottish Storytelling Centre, Edinburgh (www.scottishstorytellingcentre.co.uk) for information on training, events, clubs and networks.

The Society for Storytelling (www.sfs.org.uk) supports and promotes storytelling in England and Wales.

The International School of Storytelling, East Sussex (www.schoolofstorytelling.com) holds training courses lasting for a weekend, or for 1 – 6 weeks.

Lapidus: Creative Words for Health and Wellbeing (www.lapidus.org.uk) provides networking, workshops and courses in creative writing and arts/crafts, designed for professionals and others in the fields of Health and Wellbeing.

TALES AND TUNES

List of CD Tracks

CD 1

1. 'The Legend of Beira and Bride'
Wild Winter comp. J. Gardener
10.26

2. 'The Taen Awa'
Bad Fairy Jam comp. G. Loening
The Contented Crofters comp. G. Loening
11.35

3. 'Finn McCool and the Young Hero's Children'
20.02

4. 'The Seven Ravens'
Ruffled Feathers comp. G. Loening
10.34

5. 'The Cockerel and the Sultan'
Wild Winter comp. J. Gardener
7.28

CD 2

6. 'Jack and Marigold'
Good Old Jack comp. J. Gardener
Witch in the Woods comp. J. Gardener
17.31

7. 'One-Eye, Two-Eyes, Three-Eyes'
15.10

8. 'Tatterhood'
Sisterhood comp. J. Gardener
21.17

9. 'The Dog and the Peacock'
Warm Winter comp. J. Gardener
5.24

10. 'The Good Goodbye'
Wild Winter comp. J. Gardener
6.03

Tales written and told by Ruth Kirkpatrick

Tunes composed and played by:
Jenny Gardener – Fiddle and Guitar
Gica Loening – Fiddle, Mbira and Angklung

Engineered by David Gray at Sound Cafe www.sound-cafe.co.uk